Atlas of
Hematology

Atlas of Hematology

Shauna C. Anderson, PhD

Professor, Department of Microbiology and Molecular Biology
Brigham Young University
Provo, Utah

Keila Poulsen

Hematology Supervisor
Eastern Idaho Regional Medical Center
Idaho Falls, Idaho

 LIPPINCOTT WILLIAMS & WILKINS
A **Wolters Kluwer** Company

Philadelphia • Baltimore • New York • London
Buenos Aires • Hong Kong • Sydney • Tokyo

Editor: John Goucher
Managing Editor: Jacquelyn Merrell
Marketing Manager: Mary Martin
Production Editor: Caroline Define
Designer: Risa Clow
Compositor: TechBooks
Printer: R.R. Donnelley & Sons

351 West Camden Street
Baltimore, MD 21201

530 Walnut St.
Philadelphia, PA 19106

Printed in the United States of America

First Edition, 2003

Library of Congress Cataloging-in-Publication Data

Anderson, Shauna Christine, 1945–
  Atlas of hematology / Shauna Anderson, Keila Poulsen.
     p. ; cm.
  Includes index.
  ISBN 0-7817-2662-X
  1. Hematology—Atlases. 2. Blood—Diseases—Atlases. I. Poulsen, Keila. II. Title.
  [DNLM: 1. Hematologic Diseases—pathology—Atlases. 2. Blood
Cells—pathology—Atlases. WH 17 A549a 2002]
  RC633.A536 2002
  616.1′5′00222—dc21
                                           2002043065

To purchase additional copies of this book, call our customer service department at **(800) 638-3030** or fax orders to **(301) 824-7390**. International customers should call **(301) 714-2324**.

Visit Lippincott Williams & Wilkins on the Internet: http://www.LWW.com. Lippincott Williams & Wilkins customer service representatives are available from 8:30 am to 6:00 pm, EST.

03 04 05
1 2 3 4 5 6 7 8 9 10

Contents

Acknowledgments vii
Preface ix

UNIT I. CELL DESCRIPTIONS

Section A.   **Blood Cells** 3
Chapter 1. Red Blood Cells 3
Chapter 2. White Blood Cells 57
Chapter 3. Megakaryocytes 129
Chapter 4. Comparison of Cells 141

Section B.   **Bone Marrow** 155
Chapter 1. Cellularity 155
Chapter 2. Cells of the Reticuloendothelial System 167
Chapter 3. Nonhematopoietic Cells 173

Section C.   **Cytochemistry** 177
Chapter 1. Cytochemical Stains 177

UNIT II. HEMATOLOGIC DISORDERS

Section A.   **Red Blood Cell Disorders** 209
Chapter 1. Erythrocytosis 209
Chapter 2. Hypochromic Anemias 219
Chapter 3. Megaloblastic Anemias 253
Chapter 4. Hypoproliferative Anemias 261
Chapter 5. Qualitative Hemoglobinopathies 279
Chapter 6. Hemolytic Anemias 301
Chapter 7. Acute Blood Loss 327
Chapter 8. Anemias Associated With Systemic Disorders 331

Section B.   **White Blood Cell Disorders** 341
Chapter 1. Nonmalignant Leukocyte Disorders 341
Chapter 2. Leukemias 371
Chapter 3. Myelodysplastic Syndromes 433
Chapter 4. Myeloproliferative Diseases 453
Chapter 5. Myelodysplastic/Myeloproliferative Diseases 477
Chapter 6. Chronic Lymphoproliferative Disorders 489
Chapter 7. Lymphomas 507
Chapter 8. Plasma Cell Disorders 525

Section C.   **Miscellaneous Disorders** 537
Chapter 1. Quantitative Platelet Disorders 537
Chapter 2. Hematologic Disease Associated With Microorganisms 545
Chapter 3. Reticuloendothelial System Storage Disorders 569

Index 579

Acknowledgments

We would like to thank our families for their support because this project required an incredible time commitment.

Our students have always been a source of stimulus and enjoyment. We would like to thank them for their suggestions.

We would also like to acknowledge those individuals listed below for either providing blood smears and/or serving as reviewers of this material.

Karen A. Brown, MS, University of Utah
Fiona E. Craig, MD, University of Pittsburgh
Sarah C. Dawson, MS, King Faisal Specialist Hospital & Research Centre
Floyd Fantelli, MD, Eastern Idaho Regional Medical Center
Kristine M. Hodson, Eastern Idaho Regional Medical Center
Jean D. Holter, EdD, West Virginia University
Cheryl Jackson-Harris, MS, University of California Dominguez Hills
Amy J. Larsen, Eastern Idaho Regional Medical Center
Carol N. LeCrone, MS, University of Washington
Tim R. Randolph, MS, St. Louis University
Yasmen H. Simonian, PhD, Weber State University
Matt Tannenbaum, MD, Eastern Idaho Regional Medical Center
Jane Theobald, MS, University of Wyoming
Paul M. Urie, PhD, MD, Utah Valley Regional Medical Center
Donna Wong, MS, University of California Dominguez Hills

Many thanks to all those who have helped with this project at Lippincott Williams & Wilkins: Larry McGrew for listening to our ideas, John Goucher for assuming the project, and especially Jacqui Merrell and Rebecca R. Clark for having patience and guiding us through the process.

Shauna C. Anderson
Keila B. Poulsen

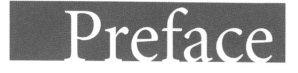

Preface

After many years of interacting with students, Shauna Anderson and Keila Poulsen have produced this atlas to accompany the interactive tools, *Anderson's Electronic Atlas of Hematology and Anderson's Electronic Atlas of Hematologic Disorders*. High-quality images are combined with in-depth descriptive text to create an ideal bench-top tool for the student and practitioner.

ORGANIZATION

The text has two units: Cell Descriptions (or normal hematology) and Hematologic Disorders. The first unit is organized into three parts:

- hematopoietic cells, including a comparison of some of the commonly confused cells
- bone marrow cellularity, cells of the reticuloendothelial system, and nonhematopoietic cells
- cytochemical stains

Each cell description includes the cell size, a description of the nucleus and cytoplasm, and a list of associated clinical conditions. A drawing of the maturation series for each cell type accompanies the high-quality photographs.

The second unit describes hematologic disorders. Each description includes a brief summary of the clinical features, pathology, laboratory features, and a diagnostic scheme. The diagnostic scheme summarizes the relevant laboratory findings that lead to the features of a particular disorder. This unit is also organized into three parts:

- red blood cell disorders, including erythrocytosis, hypochromic anemias, megaloblastic anemias, hypoproliferative anemias, qualitative hemoglobinopathies, hemolytic anemias, and acute blood loss
- white cell disorders, including nonmalignant leukocyte disorders, leukemias, myelodysplastic syndromes, myeloproliferative syndromes, myeloproliferative/myelodysplastic syndromes, chronic lymphoproliferative disorders, lymphomas, and plasma cell disorders
- miscellaneous disorders, including quantitative platelet disorders, hematologic disease associated with microorganisms, and reticuloendothelial system storage disorders

The WHO classification of hematopoietic and lymphoid tissue has been incorporated into this atlas.

IS THIS TEXT FOR YOU?

Yes! The atlas can be used to teach any level of hematology course. Whether it is used for teaching cell identification or for the diagnosis of disease, it is a valuable learning tool for students in clinical laboratory technician or clinical laboratory science programs. It is also a great reference for students in nursing and nurse practitioner programs, as well as medical students or residents. Finally, this spiral-bound atlas is an ideal, user-friendly, convenient companion at the microscope and can be used as a retraining resource or as a laboratory reference.

Unit I

Cell Descriptions

■ **Section A.** Blood Cells

■ **Section B.** Bone Marrow

■ **Section C.** Cytochemistry

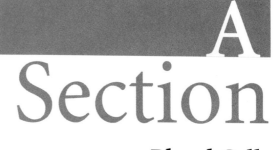

Section A

Blood Cells

CHAPTER 1

Red Blood Cells

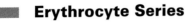

NORMAL MATURATION SERIES

Erythrocyte Series

Figure IA1-1

Pronormoblast (Rubriblast)

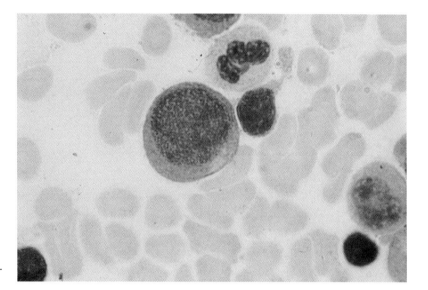

Figure **IA1-2**

Size: 14–22 μ

Nucleus

Shape: Round to slightly oval
N/C Ratio: 5:1–8:1
Color: Purple-red
Chromatin: Fine, but granular; parachromatin sparse
Nucleoli: 1–2 prominent; bluish tint

Cytoplasm

Color: Deep blue
Contents: Golgi, mitochondria, which produce a lighter blue color (perinuclear halo)

Clinical Conditions

■ Erythroleukemia (M6a)
■ Pure erythroid leukemia (M6b)
■ Hemolytic disease of the newborn

Basophilic Normoblast (Prorubricyte)

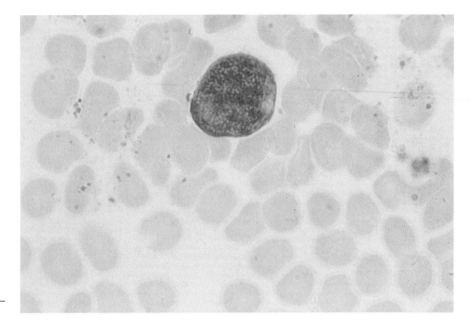

Figure **IA1-3**

Size: 12–17 μ

Nucleus

Shape: Round, centered
N/C Ratio: 4:1–6:1
Color: Purple interspersed with light areas
Chromatin: Coarse and somewhat condensed
Nucleoli: Usually not visible

Cytoplasm

Color: Deep blue
Contents: Golgi may produce a light blue area near the nucleus, many mitochondria

Clinical Conditions

- Erythroleukemia (M6a)
- Pure erythroid leukemia (M6b)
- Hemolytic disease of the newborn

Polychromatophilic Normoblast (Rubricyte)

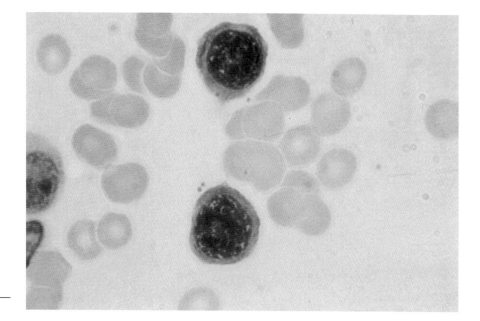

Figure **IA1-4**

Size: 11–14 μ

Nucleus

Shape: Round, centered to eccentric
N/C Ratio: 1:1–4:1
Color: Red-purple
Chromatin: Coarse and condensed; parachromatin distinct, producing a "checkerboard" appearance
Nucleoli: None

Cytoplasm

Color: Bluish-pink to grey-blue
Contents: Perinuclear halo visible; increased hemoglobin, causing the pink-grey color; decreased RNA, causing the lighter blue color

Clinical Conditions

- Erythroleukemia (M6a)
- Pure erythroid leukemia (M6b)
- Hemolytic disease of the newborn
- Myeloproliferative disease—chronic idiopathic myelofibrosis (CIMF), chronic myelocytic leukemia (CML)
- Hemolytic anemias
- Thalassemia major
- Sickle cell disease

Orthochromic Normoblast (Metarubricyte)

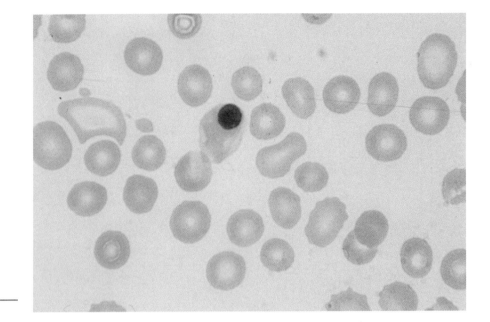

Figure IA1-5

Size: 8–12 μ

Nucleus

Shape: Round, centered to eccentric; may be fragmented or extruding
N/C Ratio: 1:4–1:2
Color: Blue-purple
Chromatin: Condensed and homogeneous (pyknotic)
Nucleoli: None

Cytoplasm

Color: Pink to orange-pink, with a hint of blue
Contents: Hemoglobin production increased

Clinical Conditions

- Erythroleukemia (M6a)
- Pure erythroid leukemia (M6b)
- Hemolytic disease of the newborn
- Myeloproliferative diseases—CIMF, CML
- Thalassemia major
- Sickle cell disease

Polychromatophilic Erythrocyte (Reticulocyte)

Figure IA1-6

Size: 8–11 μ

Nucleus

None

Cytoplasm

Color: Pink, with a tint of blue
Contents: Remnants of Golgi and mitochondria, residual RNA (reticulum)

Clinical Conditions

■ Increased erythrocyte production
■ Hemolytic anemias
■ Membrane disorders
■ Hemolytic disease of the newborn

Mature Red Blood Cell (Mature Erythrocyte)

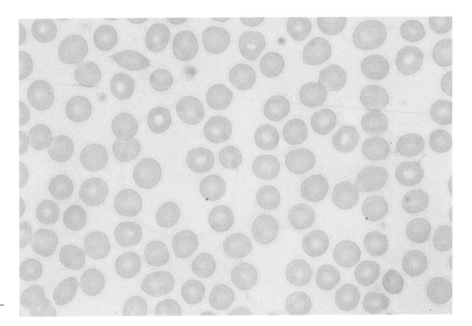

Figure IA1-7

Size: 7–7.5 μ

Nucleus

None

Cytoplasm

Color: Pink, central pallor about 1/3 of the cell
Contents: No mitochondria

MEGALOBLASTIC MATURATION SERIES

Megaloblastic Series

Figure IA1-8

Promegaloblast (Megaloblastic Rubriblast)

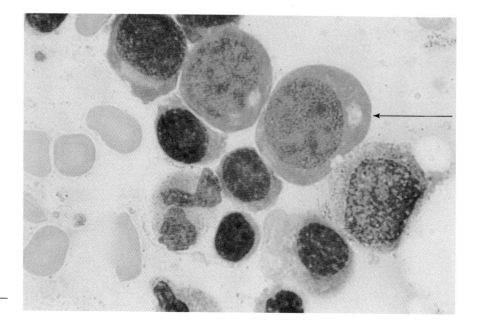

Figure IA1-9

Size: 19–27 μ

Nucleus

Shape: Round or irregular
N/C Ratio: 5:1
Color: Purple
Chromatin: Fine and closely meshed
Nucleoli: Multiple

Cytoplasm

Color: Deep blue
Contents: Nongranular with perinuclear halo

Clinical Conditions

■ Vitamin B_{12} deficiency
■ Folic acid deficiency
■ Congenital dyserythropoietic anemia

Basophilic Megaloblast (Megaloblastic Prorubricyte)

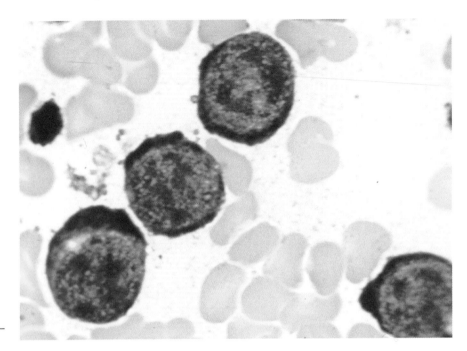

Figure **IA1-10**

Size: 17–24 μ

Nucleus

Shape: Round
N/C Ratio: 4:1
Color: Purple
Chromatin: Coarser than previous cell but still fine and open
Nucleoli: Not visible

Cytoplasm

Color: Deep blue
Contents: Faint perinuclear halo

Clinical Conditions

- Vitamin B_{12} deficiency
- Folic acid deficiency
- Congenital dyserythropoietic anemia

Polychromatophilic Megaloblast (Megaloblastic Rubricyte)

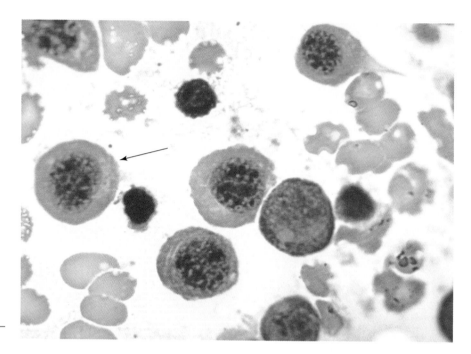

Size: 15–20 μ

Nucleus

Shape: Round and central
N/C Ratio: 2:1
Color: Purple
Chromatin: Minimal clumping, loosely defined
Nucleoli: Not visible

Cytoplasm

Color: Blue-grey to pink-grey
Contents: More cytoplasm than in normoblastic cell

Clinical Conditions

■ Vitamin B_{12} deficiency
■ Folic acid deficiency
■ Congenital dyserythropoietic anemia

Orthochromic Megaloblast (Megaloblastic Metarubricyte)

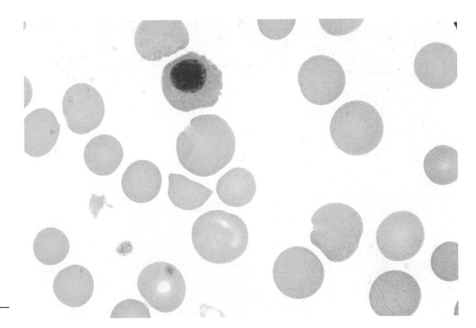

Figure IA1-12

Size: 10–15 μ

Nucleus

Shape: Round to slightly irregular, central or slightly eccentric
N/C Ratio: 1:1
Color: Deep purple but still some chromatin structure
Chromatin: Clumped, but less than in normoblastic cell
Nucleoli: Not visible

Cytoplasm

Color: Pink, with a hint of blue
Contents: More cytoplasm than in normoblastic cell

Clinical Conditions

■ Vitamin B₁₂ deficiency
■ Folic acid deficiency
■ Congenital dyserythropoietic anemia

Polychromatophilic Megalocyte (Megaloblastic Reticulocyte)

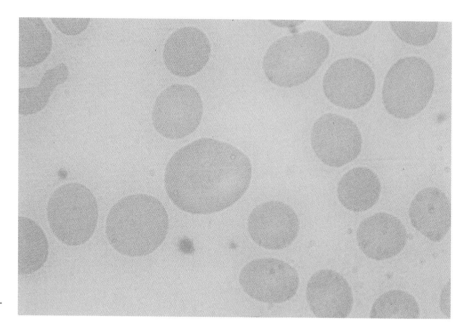

Figure IA1-13

Size: 9–15 μ

Nucleus

None

Cytoplasm

Color: Pink, with a hint of blue

Clinical Conditions

■ Vitamin B_{12} deficiency
■ Folic acid deficiency
■ Congenital dyserythropoietic anemia

Megalocyte (Oral Macrocyte)

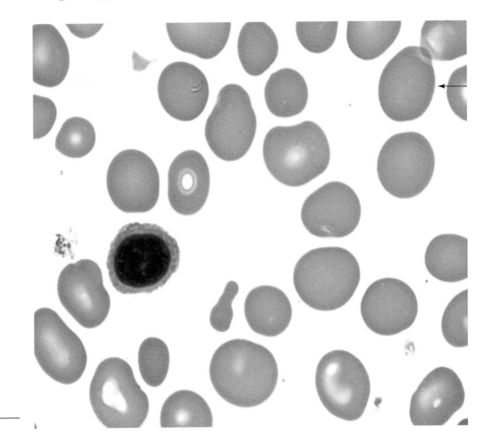

Figure IA1-14

Size: 9–12 μ

Nucleus

None

Cytoplasm

Color: Pink, central pallor less distinct
Contents: Increased hemoglobin
content

Clinical Conditions

- Vitamin B_{12} deficiency
- Folic acid deficiency
- Congenital dyserythropoietic anemia
- Myelodysplastic syndromes
- Newborn

IRON-DEFICIENT MATURATION SERIES

Iron-Deficient Series

Figure IA1-15

Iron-Deficient Pronormoblast (Iron-Deficient Rubriblast)

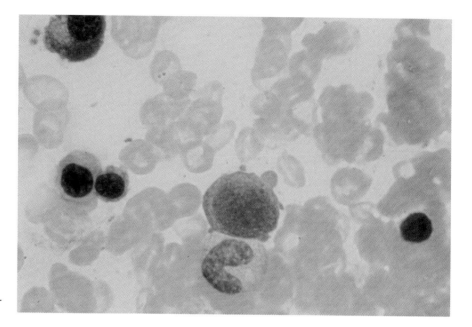

Figure IA1-16

Size: 14–20 μ

Nucleus

Shape: Irregularly round to slightly oval
N/C Ratio: 5:1
Color: Purple-red
Chromatin: Fine, but granular
Nucleoli: Present, but not distinct

Cytoplasm

Shape: Irregular
Color: Deep blue
Contents: Golgi; mitochondria, which produce a lighter blue perinuclear halo

Clinical Conditions

■ Iron deficiency
■ Anemia of chronic disease

Iron-Deficient Basophilic Normoblast (Iron-Deficient Prorubricyte)

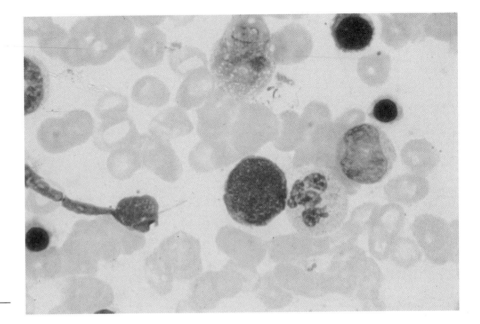

Figure IA1-17

Size: 10–15 μ

Nucleus

Shape: Round, centered
N/C Ratio: 5:1
Color: Purple, interspersed with light areas
Chromatin: Granular to slightly lumpy
Nucleoli: Usually not visible

Cytoplasm

Shape: Irregular
Color: Deep blue
Contents: Golgi may produce a light blue area near the nucleus; many mitochondria

Clinical Conditions

▪ Iron deficiency
▪ Anemia of chronic disease

Iron-Deficient Polychromatophilic Normoblast (Iron-Deficient Rubricyte)

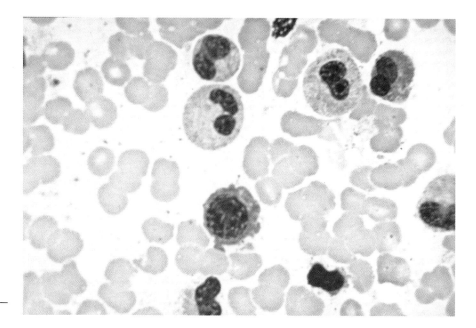

Figure IA1-18

Size: 9–12 μ

Nucleus

Shape: Round
N/C Ratio: 2:1
Color: Purple-red
Chromatin: Lumpy, with lighter parachromatin
Nucleoli: None

Cytoplasm

Color: Bluer than in normoblastic maturation
Contents: Lesser amount with shaggy blunt extensions

Clinical Conditions

■ Iron deficiency
■ Anemia of chronic disease

Iron-Deficient Orthochromic Normoblast
(Iron-Deficient Metarubricyte)

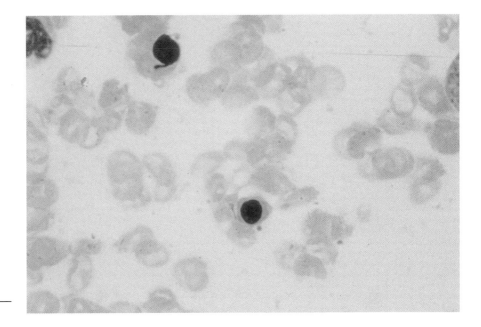

Figure **IA1-19**

Size: 7–11 μ

Nucleus

Shape: Round
N/C Ratio: 1:2
Color: Blue-purple
Chromatin: Condensed and homogeneous
Nucleoli: None

Cytoplasm

Shape: Irregular
Color: Pink, with residual blueness of RNA

Clinical Conditions

■ Iron deficiency
■ Anemia of chronic diseases

Iron-Deficient Polychromatophilic Erythrocyte

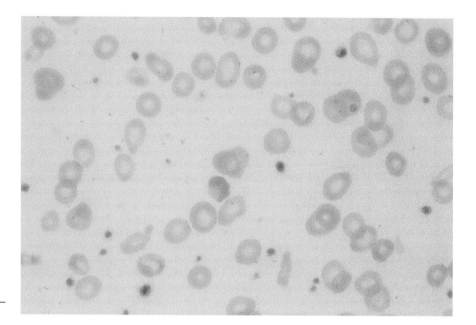

Figure **IA1-20**

Size: **<6.5–10** μ

Nucleus

None

Cytoplasm

Color: Pink, with a hint of blue

Clinical Conditions

■ Iron deficiency
■ Anemia of chronic diseases

Iron-Deficient Erythrocyte (Hypochromic/Microcytic)

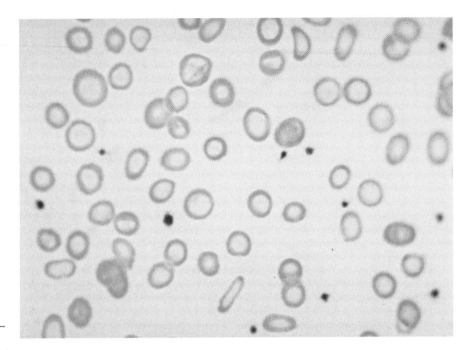

Figure IA1-21

Size: <6.5 μ

Nucleus

None

Cytoplasm

Color: Pink, central pallor greater than one-third of cell
Contents: Hemoglobin decreased

Clinical Conditions

■ Iron deficiency
■ Anemia of chronic disease

DISTRIBUTION

Agglutination

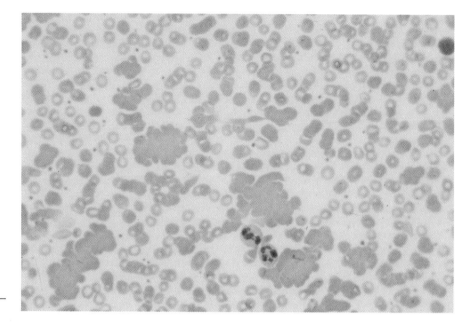

Figure **IA1-22**

Cell Type

Mature red blood cells

Description

Random masses or clusters of cells

Clinical Conditions

- Exposure to a variety of antibodies
- Hemolytic anemia (autoimmune)
- Atypical pneumonia
- Staphylococcal infections
- Trypanosomiasis
- Cold agglutinin disease

Rouleaux

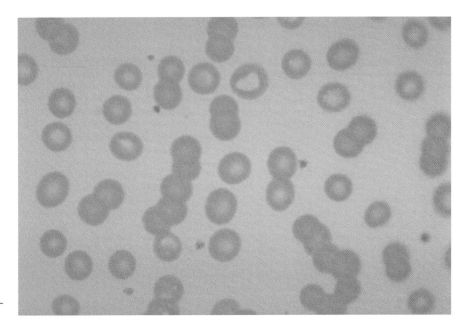

Cell Type

Mature red blood cell

Description

Short or long stacks of cells (three or four or more) resembling coins; often a
blue-staining background is also present

Clinical Conditions

■ Hyperproteinemia
■ Multiple myeloma
■ Macroglobulinemia
■ Increased fibrinogen (infection, pregnancy)

SHAPES

Acanthocyte

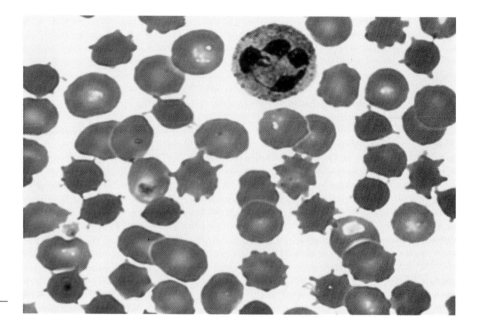

Figure **IA1-24**

Cell Type

Mature red blood cell

Description

Spherical and densely stained cell with 3–12 spicules of uneven length and width around the surface

Clinical Conditions

- Inherited lipid disorder (abetalipoproteinemia)
- Alcoholic cirrhosis
- Malabsorption states
- Neonatal hepatitis
- Pyruvate kinase deficiency

Codocyte (Target Cell)

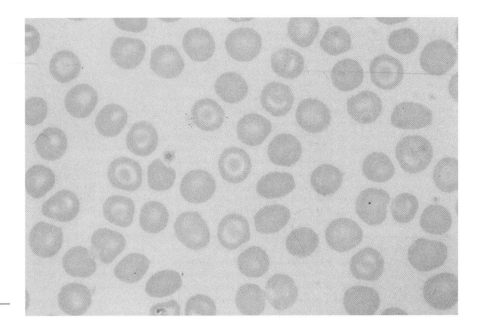

Figure IA1-25

Cell Type

Mature red blood cell

Description

Bell shaped, with a thin wall having a greater-than-normal surface membrane:volume ratio; central area of hemoglobin, a clear ring, and a peripheral ring of hemoglobin, giving an appearance of a bull's eye

Clinical Conditions

■ Hemoglobinopathies
■ Thalassemia
■ Obstructive liver disease
■ Iron deficiency anemia

Dacryocyte (Teardrop Cell)

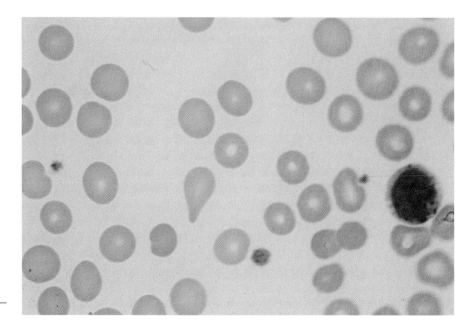

Cell Type

Mature red blood cell

Description

Pear-shaped cell with a blunt pointed projection

Clinical Conditions

- Extramedullary hematopoiesis (myelofibrosis, myelophthisic anemia)
- Megaloblastic anemia
- Thalassemia
- Hypersplenism
- Renal disease

Degmacyte (Bite Cell)

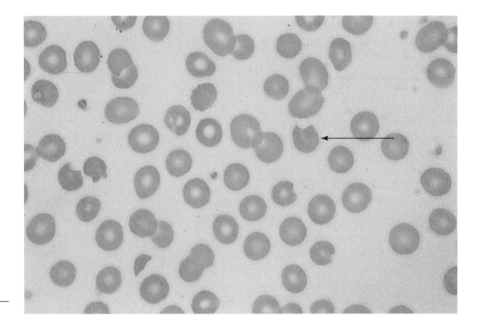

Figure IA1-27

Cell Type

Mature red blood cell

Description

Semicircular area (denatured and precipitated masses of hemoglobin) of cell
removed by spleen; these cells may show multiple peripheral defects

Clinical Conditions

■ Drug-induced anemias
■ Glucose-6-phosphate dehydrogenase deficiency
■ Thalassemia
■ Unstable hemoglobinopathies

Drepanocyte (Sickle Cell)

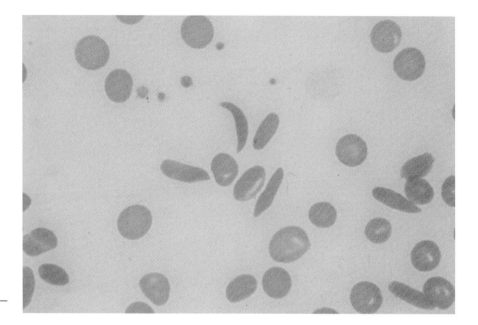

Figure **IA1-28**

Cell Type

Mature red blood cell

Description

Elongated cell due to polymers of abnormal hemoglobin; terminal projections, causing the cell to take on an irregular shape; usually lacks a central pallor

Clinical Conditions

■ Hemoglobinopathies (SS, SC, SD, S-β thalassemia)

Echinocyte (Burr Cell)

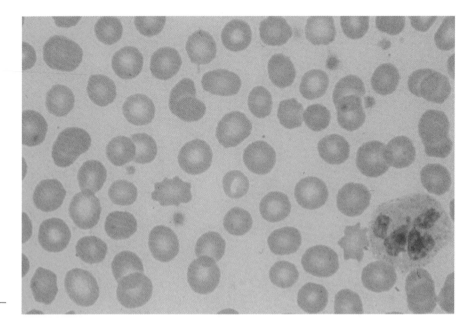

Figure IA1-29

Cell Type

Mature red blood cell

Description

Cell with evenly distributed, short spicules; the spicules have a blunt end; retains
  central pallor

Clinical Conditions

■ Slow drying in high humidity
■ Renal insufficiency
■ Pyruvate kinase deficiency
■ Stored blood
■ Severe dehydration
■ Burns

Keratocyte (Horn Cell)

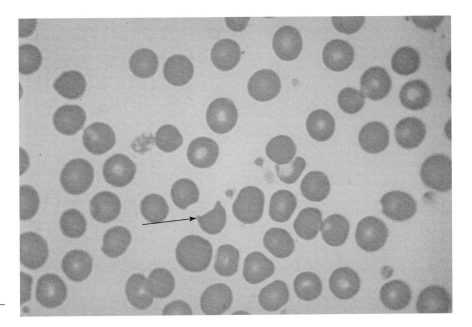

Figure IA1-30

Cell Type

Mature red blood cell

Description

Cell with projections (usually two) that resemble horns

Clinical Conditions

■ Microangiopathic hemolytic anemia
■ Glomerulonephritis
■ Waring Blender syndrome
■ Pyruvate kinase deficiency

Knizocyte (Pinch Cell)

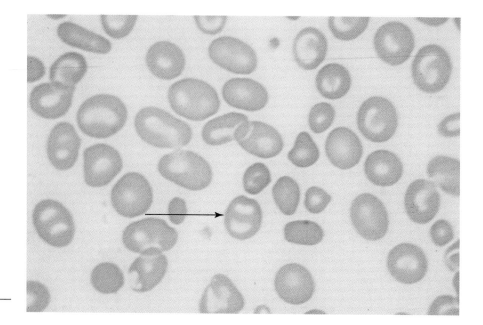

Figure IA1-31

Cell Type

Mature red blood cell

Description

Cell with triconcave shape having two central pallors

Clinical Conditions

■ Hemolytic anemia
■ Hemoglobinopathies
■ Pancreatitis

Ovalocyte (Elliptocyte)

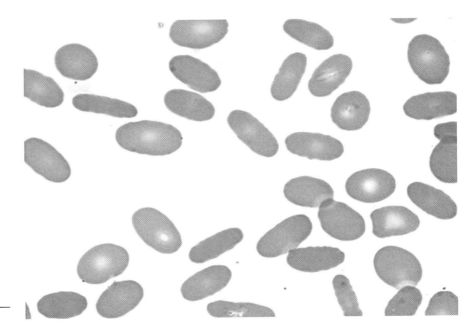

Figure IA1-32

Cell Type

Mature red blood cell

Description

Oval-shaped cell (may be slightly egg, rod, or pencil shaped); hemoglobin is concentrated at two ends; normal central pallor

Clinical Conditions

■ Hereditary elliptocytosis
■ Iron deficiency anemia
■ Myelophthisic anemia
■ Megaloblastic anemia
■ Thalassemia
■ Sideroblastic anemia
■ Congenital dyserythropoietic anemia

Pyknocyte (Blister Cell)

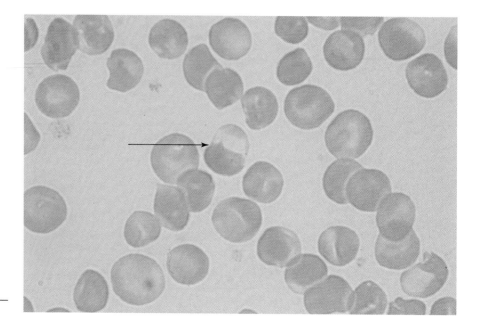

Cell Type

Mature red blood cell

Description

Cell with a clearing on one side and a concentrated area of hemoglobin on the other side

Clinical Conditions

■ Infantile pyknocytosis
■ Infantile viremia

Schistocyte (Schizocyte)

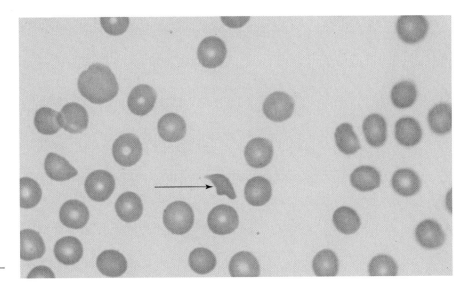

Figure IA1-34

Cell Type

Mature red blood cell

Description

Irregular shape or fragment of cell; results from damaged membrane

Clinical Conditions

■ Microangiopathic hemolytic anemias
■ Traumatic hemolytic anemias
■ Waring Blender syndrome

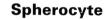

Spherocyte

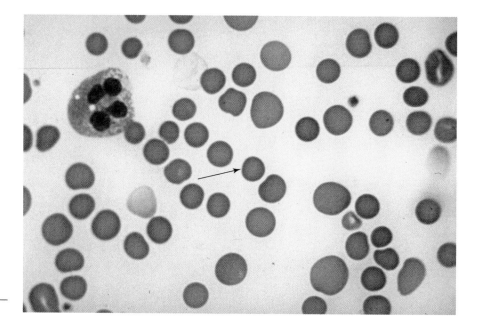

Cell Type

Mature red blood cell

Size: 6.1–7.0 μ

Description

Round cells; increased staining intensity with no central pallor; smaller volume than a normal cell (decreased surface:volume ratio)

Clinical Conditions

- Hereditary spherocytosis
- Immunohemolytic anemias
- Heinz body hemolytic anemia
- Severe burns (microspherocytes seen); microspherocytes are <4.0 μ
- Hypersplenism

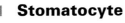

Stomatocyte

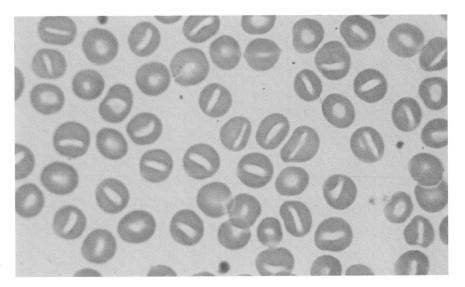

Figure IA1-36

Cell Type

Mature red blood cell

Description

Cell having a slitlike area of central pallor

Clinical Conditions

■ Hereditary stomatocytosis
■ Alcoholism
■ Obstructive liver disease
■ Cirrhosis
■ Rh-null disease

Macrocyte

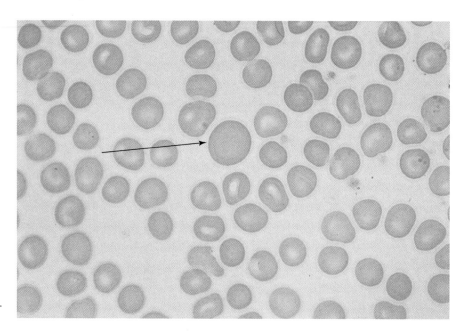

Figure IA1-37

Size: >7.8 μ

Cell Type

Mature red blood cell

Description

Large cell, mean corpuscular volume usually >100 fL; usually normochromic; may be round or oval; cytoplasm is pink-red

Clinical Conditions

■ Liver disease (round macrocytes seen)
■ Megaloblastic anemias (oval macrocytes seen)
■ Myelodysplastic syndrome
■ Acute blood loss
■ Chemotherapy

Microcyte

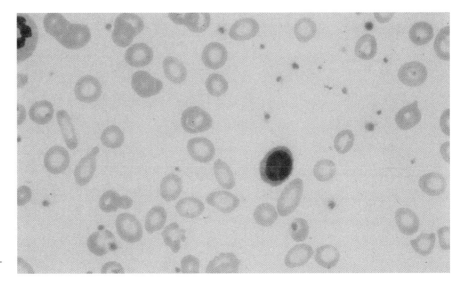

Figure IA1-38

Size: $< 6.5\ \mu$

Cell Type

Mature red blood cell

Description

Smaller than a normal cell; mean corpuscular volume usually <80 fL; has a central
pallor; normochromic or hypochromic

Clinical Conditions

- Iron deficiency anemia
- Thalassemias
- Lead poisoning
- Anemia of chronic disease
- Sideroblastic anemia

COLORING

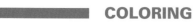

Dimorphic

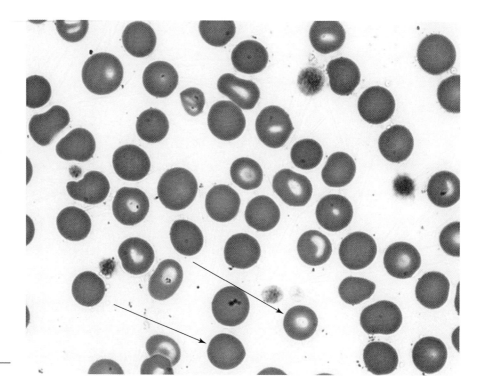

Figure IA1-39

Cell Type

Mature erythrocytes

Size: 6–11 μ

Description

Dual population of cells, normocytic and microcytic; normocytic and macrocytic;
may also exhibit normochromia and hypochromia

Clinical Conditions

■ Sideroblastic anemia
■ Myelodysplastic syndromes

Hypochromic

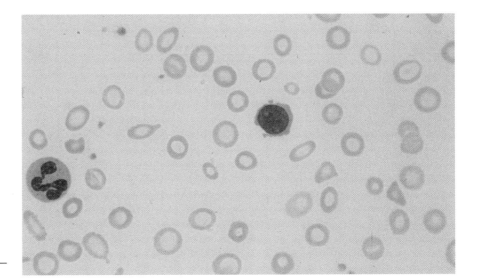

Figure **IA1-40**

Cell Type

Mature red blood cell

Description

Cells possess a greater central pallor than normal (greater than one-third); may lack hemoglobin and have a decreased mean corpuscular hemoglobin concentration or may be abnormally thin

Clinical Conditions

■ Iron deficiency anemia
■ Thalassemia
■ Anemia of chronic disease
■ Sideroblastic anemia
■ Myelodysplastic syndromes

Polychromatophilic

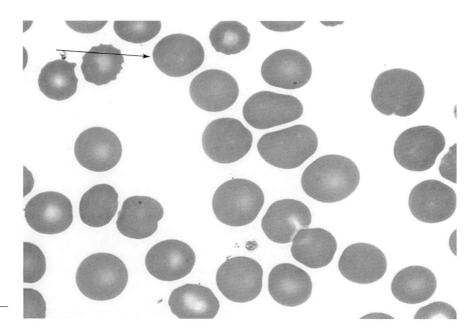

Cell Type

Young red blood cell with no nucleus

Size: 8–11 μ

Description

Contains residual RNA, which stains diffusely blue; identified as reticulocyte when stained with a supravital dye

Clinical Conditions

- Increased erythrocyte production
- Hemolytic anemias
- Membrane disorders
- Hemolytic disease of the newborn

INCLUSIONS

Basophilic Stippling (Punctuate Basophilia)

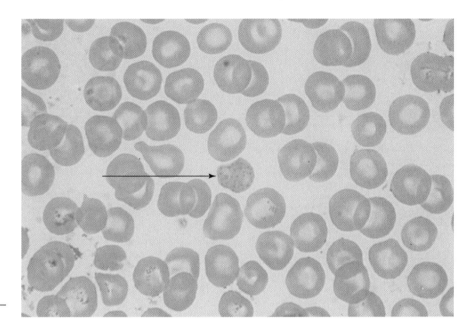

Figure IA1-42

Cell Type

Mature red blood cell

Description

Coarse, deep blue inclusions; irregularly aggregated or clumped ribosomes
throughout the cell; mitochondria and siderosomes may also aggregate

Clinical Conditions

■ Altered hemoglobin biosynthesis
■ Lead intoxication
■ Thalassemia
■ Megaloblastic anemia
■ Alcoholism
■ Sideroblastic anemia
■ Pyrimidine-5′-nucleotidase deficiency

Cabot Ring

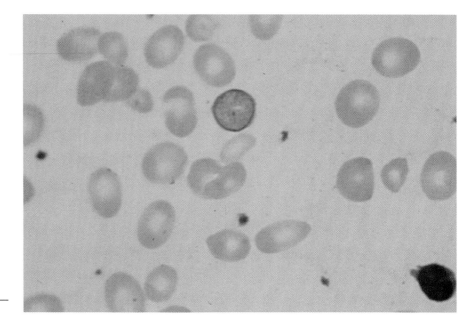

Cell Type

Mature red blood cell

Description

Oval or figure eight–shaped inclusion; red-violet; usually one per cell; consists of
   nuclear remnants or part of the mitotic spindle

Clinical Conditions

■ Severe anemias
■ Dyserythropoiesis

Heinz Bodies

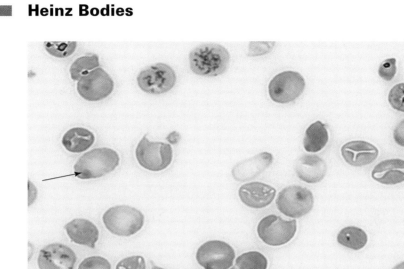

Figure IA1-44

Cell Type

Young and mature red blood cells

Size: 1–2 μ

Description

Round, refractile inclusions found on the periphery of the cell when stained with a supravital dye; consists of denatured globin produced by the destruction of hemoglobin; they may occur in multiple numbers

Clinical Conditions

■ Drug-induced anemias
■ Thalassemia
■ Glucose-6-phosphate dehydrogenase deficiency and other red blood cell enzymopathies
■ Unstable hemoglobinopathies

Hemoglobin C Crystals

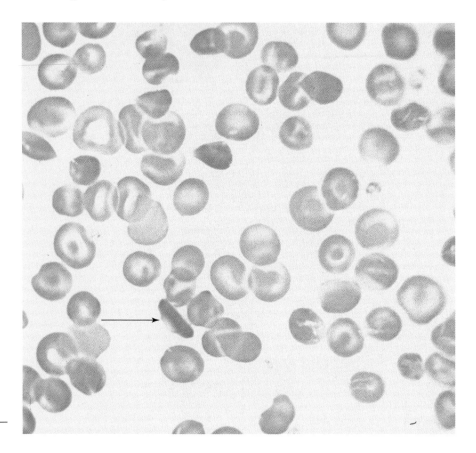

Cell Type

Mature red blood cells

Description

Hexagonal, rod-shaped inclusions with blunt ends that stain very dark; formed
within the cell membrane; remainder of cell has a clear area

Clinical Condition

■ Hemoglobin CC disease

Hemoglobin H Inclusions

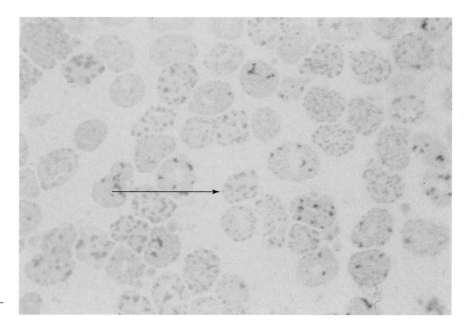

Figure IA1-46

Cell Type

Nucleated and nonnucleated red blood cells

Description

Unpaired beta-chains form small, greenish-blue inclusions when stained with
brilliant cresyl blue; uniformly dispersed throughout the cell; when present in
multiple numbers, they give the cell a "golf ball" appearance

Clinical Condition

▪ Hemoglobin H disease

Hemoglobin SC Crystals

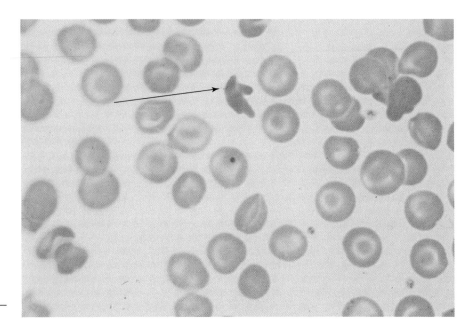

Figure IA1-47

Cell Type

Mature red blood cell

Description

Darkly stained condensed hemoglobin; crystals may be straight with parallel sides and a blunt protruding end or have several fingerlike projections from the center; crystals may protrude from the cell membrane; remainder of cell has pallor or distorted membrane

Clinical Condition

■ Hemoglobin SC disease

■ **Howell-Jolly Body**

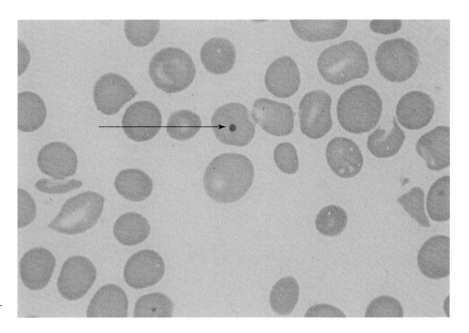

Figure IA1-48

Size: 0.5–1.0 μ

Cell Type

Nucleated and nonnucleated red blood cells

Description

Round fragments of nucleus (DNA); reddish-blue to deep purple; usually one per
  cell but occasionally may be two or more; represents chromosomes that have
  been separated from the mitotic spindle during abnormal mitosis; may also
  appear to arise from nuclear fragmentation or abnormal expulsion of the nucleus

Clinical Conditions

■ Megaloblastic anemia
■ Hemolytic anemias
■ Hyposplenism
■ Splenectomized persons
■ Alcoholism
■ Sickle cell anemia

Malaria

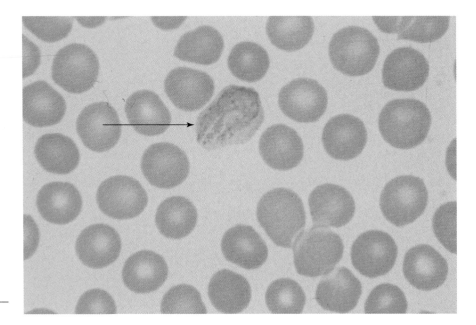

Figure IA1-49

Cell Type

Red blood cell

Description

Depends on the species of *Plasmodium* that infects the cells:

Plasmodium vivax infection enlarges the cell; Schüffner's granules may be present
Plasmodium malariae infection does not enlarge the cell
Plasmodium falciparum infection produces delicate ring forms; cells are not
enlarged; Schüffner's granules are not present
Plasmodium ovale infection produces large, oval cells; Schüffner's granules are
present

Clinical Conditions

■ *Plasmodium* infections

Pappenheimer Body

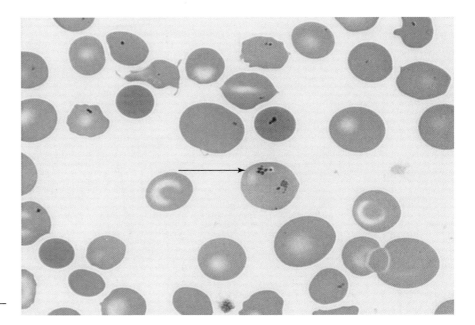

Figure IA1-50

Cell Type

Mature red blood cells, reticulocytes, metarubricytes

Description

Small, irregular, pale blue– to dark-staining granules; usually found on the periphery of the cell and in groups; smaller than Howell-Jolly bodies; represent siderosomes, which stain positive with Perls' Prussian blue stain and indicate iron content

Clinical Conditions

- Disturbed hemoglobin synthesis
- Sideroblastic anemia
- Dyserythropoietic anemias
- Thalassemia
- Myelodysplastic syndromes

ABNORMAL MATURATION

Dyserythropoiesis

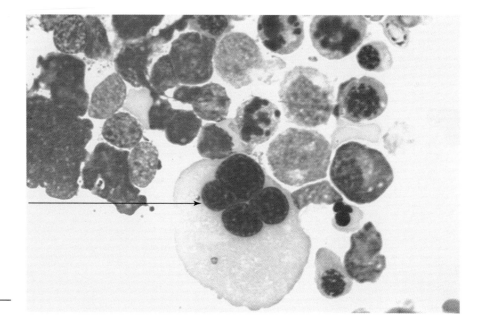

Figure IA1-51

Cell Type

Red blood cell precursors

Description

Abnormal findings in red blood cell precursors, including abnormal nuclear shapes, more than one nucleus, nuclear fragments, megaloblastoid and/or megaloblastic maturation, and vacuolated cytoplasm

Clinical Conditions

■ Myelodysplastic syndromes
■ Megaloblastic anemias
■ Erythroleukemia (M6a)
■ Pure erythroid leukemia (M6b)
■ Arsenic poisoning

CHAPTER

2

White Blood Cells

NORMAL GRANULOCYTIC MATURATION SERIES

Neutrophilic Series

Figure IA2-1

Eosinophilic Series

Basophilic Series

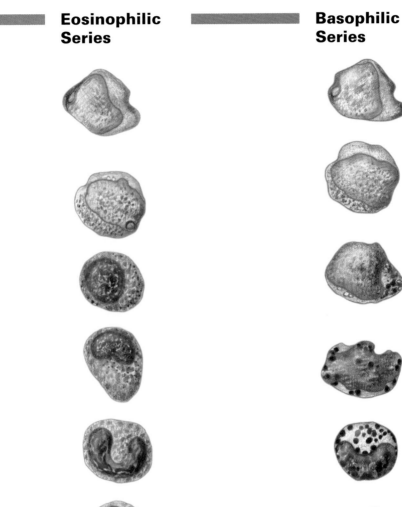

Figure IA2-2

Figure IA2-3

Myeloblast

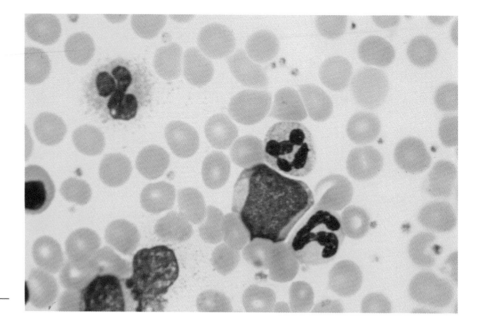

Size: 15–20 μ

Nucleus

Shape: Round
N/C Ratio: 7:1–4:1
Color: Reddish-purple
Chromatin: Delicate and dispersed
Nucleoli: 2–3

Cytoplasm

Color: Pale to deep blue; lighter staining adjacent to nucleus
Contents: Varying amounts of granules depending on whether the blast is classified as Type I, II, or III

Clinical Conditions

■ Myelodysplastic syndromes—refractory anemia with excess blasts (RAEB) 1, RAEB 2
■ Myeloproliferative diseases—CML, CIMF
■ Acute myelocytic leukemia minimally differentiated (M0)
■ Acute myelocytic leukemia without maturation (M1)
■ Acute myelocytic leukemia with maturation (M2)
■ Acute promyelocytic leukemia (M3)
■ Acute myelomonocytic leukemia (M4)
■ Erythroleukemia (M6a)
■ Acute myelocytic leukemia with multilineage dysplasia
■ Acute monoblastic leukemia (M5a)—minimal population of myeloblasts
■ Acute monocytic leukemia (M5b)—minimal population of myeloblasts

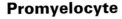

Promyelocyte

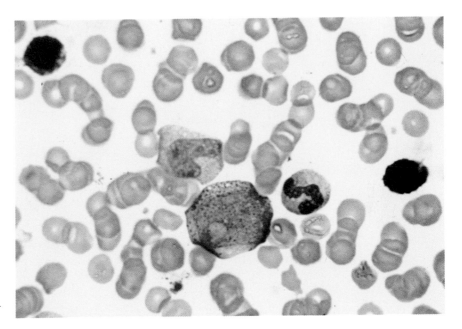

Size:18–25 μ

Nucleus

Shape: Round or oval; central or eccentric
N/C Ratio: 2:1–5:1
Color: Purple
Chromatin: Relatively fine, becoming coarser
Nucleoli: 2–3, varying from visible to indistinct

Cytoplasm

Color: Blue; lighter staining adjacent to nucleus
Contents: Few to many dark blue or reddish-blue primary granules

Clinical Conditions

- Acute myelocytic leukemia with maturation (M2)
- Acute promyelocytic leukemia (M3)
- Myeloproliferative diseases—CML, CIMF
- Growth factor therapy
- Severe infections
- Acute myelomonocytic leukemia (M4)
- Erythroleukemia (M6a)
- Pure erythroid leukemia (M6b)
- Acute myelocytic leukemia with multilineage dysplasia

Neutrophilic Myelocyte

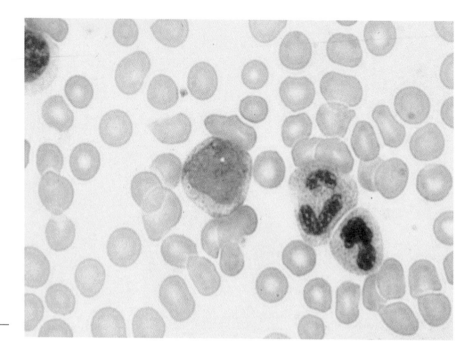

Figure IA2-6

Size: 12–18 μ

Nucleus

Shape: Round, oval, or flattened on one side
N/C Ratio: 3:1–3:2
Color: Dark purple
Chromatin: Coarser chromatin pattern
Nucleoli: Early myelocytes may have visible nucleoli

Cytoplasm

Color: Pinkish-blue
Contents: Variable numbers of nonspecific granules; small, pinkish to reddish specific granules first appearing next to the nucleus and then throughout the cytoplasm

Clinical Conditions

■ Acute myelocytic leukemia with maturation (M2)
■ Growth factor therapy
■ Myeloproliferative diseases—CML, CIMF
■ Stress
■ Severe infections

Eosinophilic Myelocyte

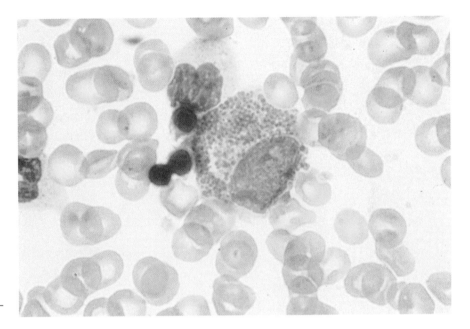

Figure IA2-7

Size: 12–18 μ

Nucleus

Shape: Round, oval, or flattened on one side
N/C Ratio: 3:1–3:2
Color: Dark purple
Chromatin: Courser chromatin pattern
Nucleoli: Early myelocytes may have visible nucleoli

Cytoplasm

Color: Pinkish-blue
Contents: Numerous large, round specific granules staining orange-brown to orange-blue; variable numbers of nonspecific granules

Clinical Conditions

■ Chronic eosinophilic leukemia
■ Hypereosinophilic syndrome

BASOPHILIC MYELOCYTE

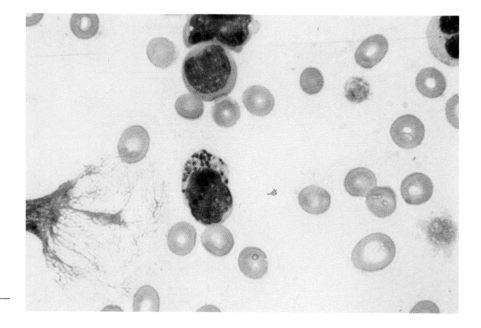

Figure IA2-8

Size: 12–18 μ

Nucleus

Shape: Round, oval, or flattened on one side
N/C Ratio: 3:1–3:2
Color: Dark purple
Chromatin: Coarser chromatin pattern
Nucleoli: Early myelocytes may have visible nucleoli

Cytoplasm

Color: Pinkish-blue
Contents: Few large specific granules staining dark bluish–purple to bluish-black

Clinical Conditions

■ Acute basophilic leukemia

Neutrophilic Metamyelocyte

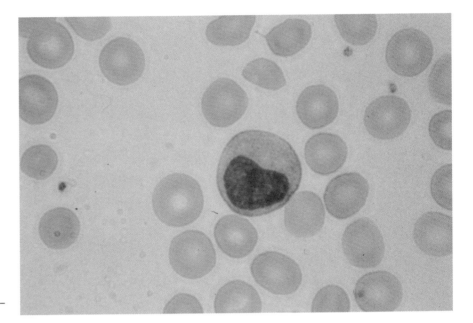

Figure IA2-9

Size: 10–15 μ

Nucleus

Shape: Typical kidney shape or slightly indented
N/C Ratio: 7:3–1:1
Color: Dark purple
Chromatin: Coarse, blue-black chromatin
Nucleoli: None

Cytoplasm

Color: Pink-blue
Contents: Pinkish to reddish-blue granules

Eosinophilic Metamyelocyte

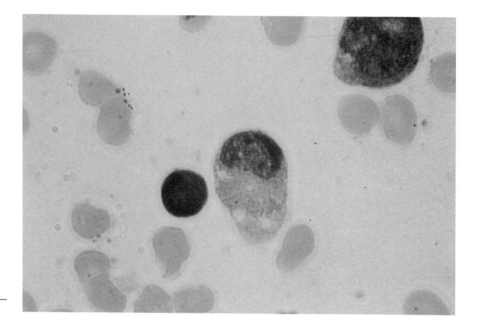

Figure IA2-10

Size: 10–15 μ

Nucleus

Shape: Typical kidney shape or slightly indented
N/C Ratio: 7:3–1:1
Color: Dark purple
Chromatin: Coarse blue-black
Nucleoli: None

Cytoplasm

Color: Pink-blue
Contents: Numerous medium bright orange to reddish granules

Basophilic Metamyelocyte

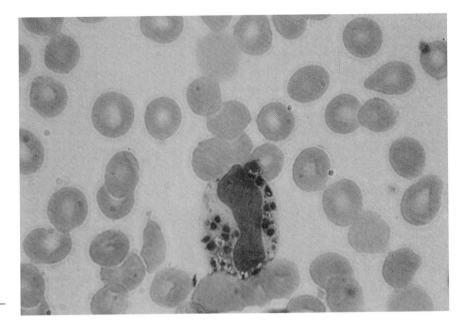

Figure IA2-11

Size: 10–15 μ

Nucleus

Shape: Typical kidney shape or slightly indented
N/C Ratio: 7:3–1:1
Color: Dark purple
Chromatin: Coarse, blue-black
Nucleoli: None

Cytoplasm

Color: Pink-blue
Contents: Few large dark blue–black granules

Neutrophilic Band

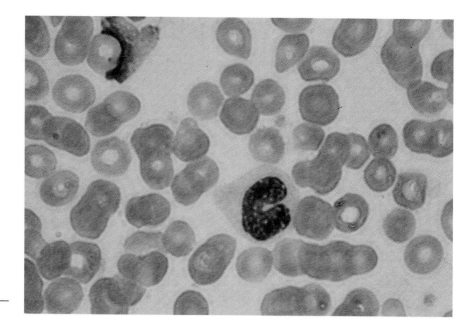

Size: 10–16 μ

Nucleus

Shape: Band shaped or markedly indented; indentation is greater than one-half the
width of the hypothetical round nucleus
N/C Ratio: 1:1–1:2
Color: Dark purple
Chromatin: Coarse, blue-black

Cytoplasm

Color: Pink-blue
Contents: Pinkish-blue granules

Eosinophilic Band

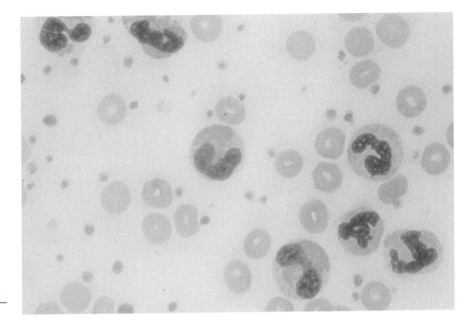

Figure IA2-13

Size: 10–16 μ

Nucleus

Shape: Band shaped or markedly indented
N/C Ratio: 1:1–1:2
Color: Dark purple
Chromatin: Coarse, blue-black
Nucleoli: None

Cytoplasm

Color: Pink-blue
Contents: Numerous orange-red granules

Basophilic Band

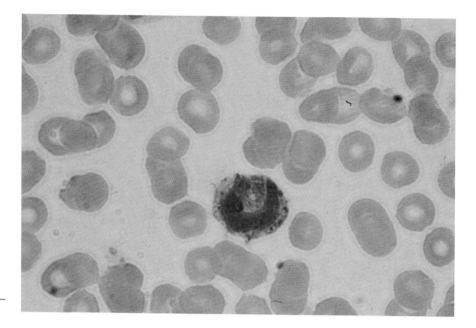

Figure **IA2-14**

Size: 10–16 μ

Nucleus

Shape: Band shaped or markedly indented
N/C Ratio: 1:1–1:2
Color: Dark purple
Chromatin: Coarse, blue-black
Nucleoli: None

Cytoplasm

Color: Pink-blue
Contents: Few large dark bluish–purple to bluish-black granules

Segmented Neutrophil (Polymorphonuclear Neutrophil)

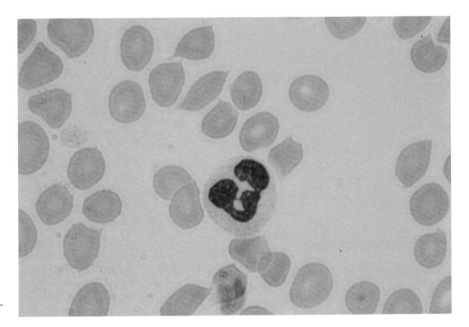

Figure IA2-15

Size: 10–16 μ

Nucleus

Shape: 2–5 lobes connected by a very narrow filament; nuclear indentation is greater than one-half its diameter
N/C Ratio: 1:3–1:5
Color: Dark purple
Chromatin: Heavily clumped
Nucleoli: None

Cytoplasm

Color: Light pink to bluish
Contents: Many small, evenly distributed pink to rose-violet granules

Clinical Conditions

■ Infections
■ Chronic neutrophilic leukemia
■ Growth factor therapy

Eosinophil

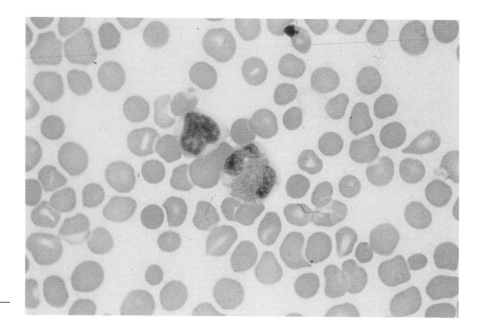

Figure IA2-16

Size: 10–16 μ

Nucleus

Shape: 2–3 lobes
N/C Ratio: 1:3–1:5
Color: Dark purple
Chromatin: Heavily clumped
Nucleoli: None

Cytoplasm

Color: Pink-blue
Contents: Many large, round, uniform reddish-orange granules

Clinical Conditions

- Protozoan infections
- Hypereosinophilic syndrome
- Allergic disorders
- Chronic myelocytic leukemia
- Dermatitis
- Hodgkin lymphoma

Basophil

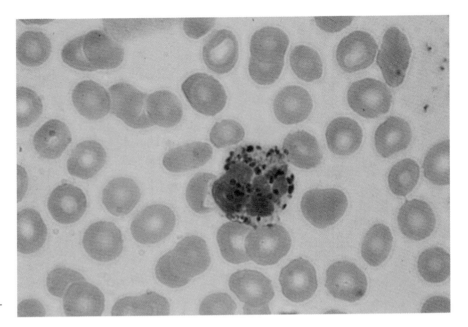

Figure IA2-17

Size: 10–16 μ

Nucleus

Shape: 2 lobes usually obscured by granules
N/C Ratio: 1:3–1:5
Color: Dark purple
Chromatin: Heavily clumped
Nucleoli: None

Cytoplasm

Color: Pink-blue
Contents: Few dark blue–black granules

Clinical Conditions

■ Acute basophilic leukemia
■ Myeloproliferative diseases
■ Allergy and inflammation
■ Infection—chicken pox

Mast Cell

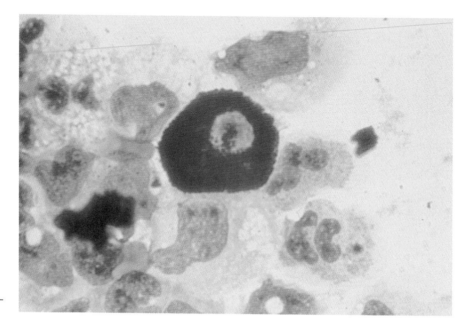

Size: 9–12 μ

Nucleus

Shape: Round
N/C Ratio: 1:1
Color: Dark purple
Chromatin: Heavily clumped
Nucleoli: None

Cytoplasm

Color: Dark blue
Contents: Many dark blue granules

Clinical Conditions

▪ Mast cell disease

NUCLEAR SEGMENTATION

Hypersegmentation

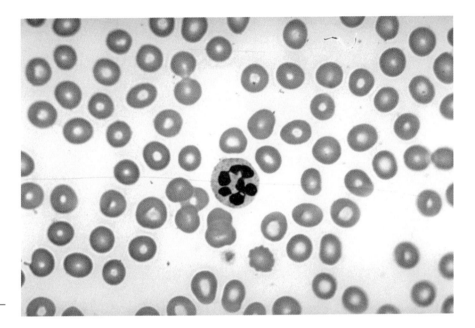

Cell Type

Neutrophil, eosinophil

Description

Neutrophil has six or more nuclear lobes; eosinophil has greater than four lobes

Clinical Conditions

■ Chronic infections
■ B$_{12}$ deficiency
■ Folic acid deficiency
■ Myelodysplastic syndromes
■ Hereditary hypersegmentation
■ Long-term infections

Pelger-Huët

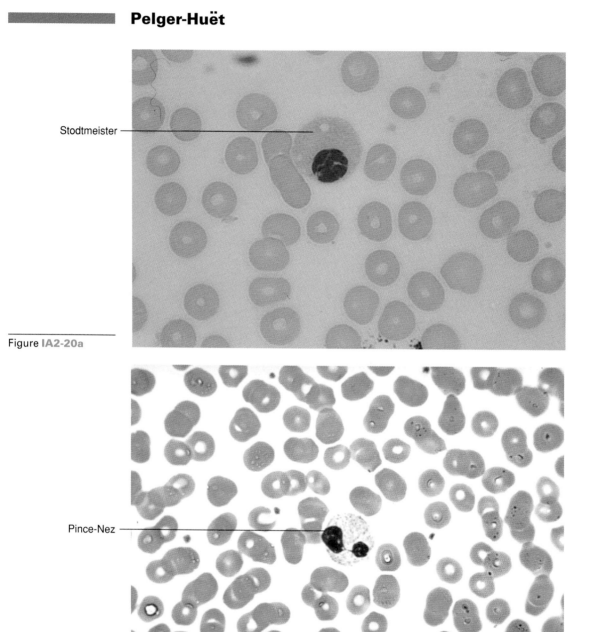

Stodtmeister

Figure IA2-20a

Pince-Nez

Figure IA2-20b

Cell Type

Neutrophil

Description

Heterozygous inherited disorder (Pince-Nez)
Bilobed or dumbbell-shaped nucleus; clumped, coarse chromatin; normal
cytoplasmic granules
Homozygous inherited disorder (Stodtmeister)
Round or oval nuclei; dense clumped coarse chromatin; normal cytoplasmic
granules

Clinical Conditions

■ Pelger-Huët—inherited disorder (autosomal dominant)

Pelgeroid Cells

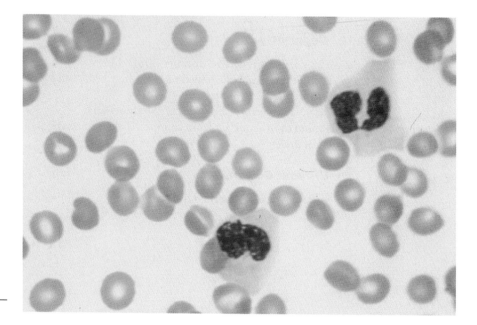

Cell Type

Neutrophil

Description

Nucleus resembles Pelger-Huët (round or bilobed); few or no cytoplasmic granules

Clinical Conditions

- Myelodysplastic syndromes
- Acute nonlymphocytic leukemias (acute myelogenous leukemias)—dysplastic finding
- Myelodysplastic/myeloproliferative diseases

CYTOPLASMIC INCLUSIONS

Alder-Reilly Bodies

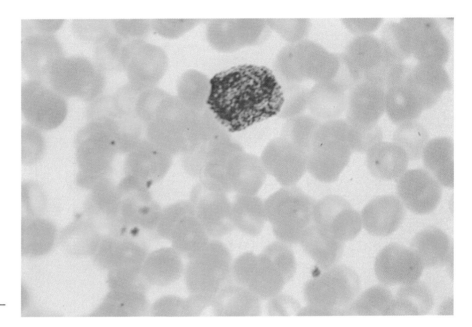

Figure IA2-22

Cell Type

Neutrophil, eosinophil, basophil; occasionally lymphocyte and monocyte

Description

Inherited condition (autosomal recessive)
Dense blue cytoplasmic granules consisting of stored mucopolysaccharides and
    sphingomyelin
Normal nuclear maturation

Clinical Conditions

■ Mucopolysaccharidoses (e.g., Hurler's syndrome, Hunter's syndrome)

Auer Rods

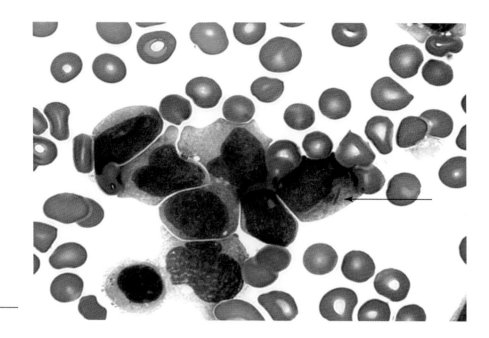

Cell Type

Myeloblast and monoblast (rare)

Description

Reddish-purple, rod-shaped cytoplasmic inclusions
Alignment of primary granules

Clinical Conditions

- Acute myelocytic leukemia without maturation (M1)
- Acute myelocytic leukemia with maturation (M2)
- Acute promyelocytic leukemia (M3)
- Acute myelomonocytic leukemia (M4)
- Erythroleukemia (M6a)
- Acute myelocytic leukemia with multilineage dysplasia
- Chronic myelocytic leukemia in blastic transformation

Chédiak-Higashi Granules

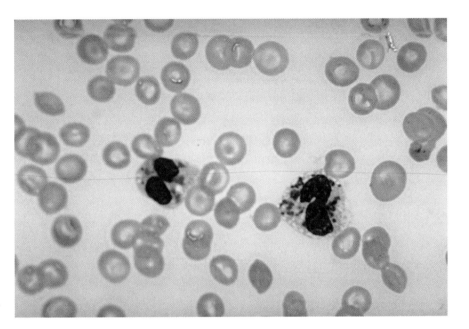

Figure IA2-24

Cell Type

Granulocyte, lymphocyte, monocyte

Description

Inherited (autosomal recessive)
Many large, greenish primary cytoplasmic granules or many large, reddish-purple
  secondary cytoplasmic granules

Clinical Conditions

■ Chédiak-Higashi Syndrome—severe and often fatal infections in children;
  complete or partial albinism

Döhle Body

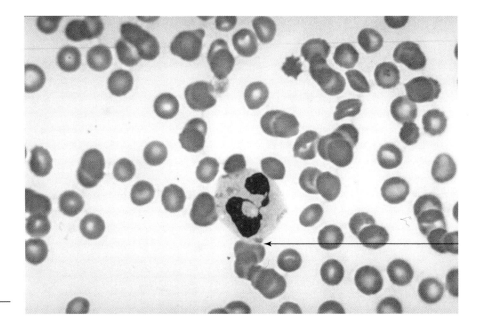

Cell Type

Neutrophil, eosinophil, basophil, monocyte

Description

Round or rod-shaped, light-blue cytoplasmic inclusions, often located near cell
   membrane
Inclusions represent ribosomes or rough endoplasmic reticulum

Clinical Conditions

- Infections
- Drug intoxication
- Burns
- Myelodysplastic syndromes, often seen in the degranulated segmented cells
- May-Hegglin anomaly
- Pregnancy
- Growth factor therapy

Faggot Cell

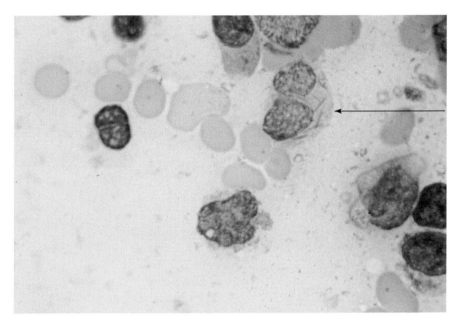

Cell Type

Promyelocyte

Description

Groups or stacks of cigar-shaped rods in cytoplasm

Clinical Conditions

■ Acute promyelocytic leukemia (M3, M3v)

May-Hegglin Inclusion

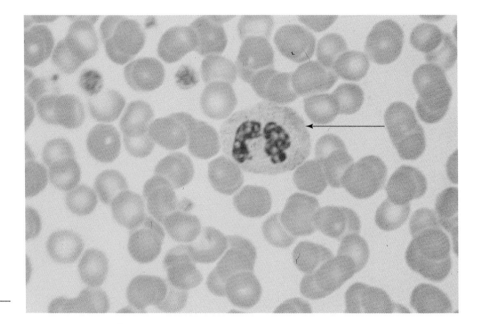

Figure IA2-27

Cell Type

Neutrophil, eosinophil, basophil, monocyte

Description

Inherited (autosomal dominant)
Large, blue, crescent-shaped cytoplasmic inclusions consisting of RNA
Resemble large Döhle bodies
Presence of enlarged platelets

Clinical Conditions

■ May-Hegglin anomaly

Microorganisms

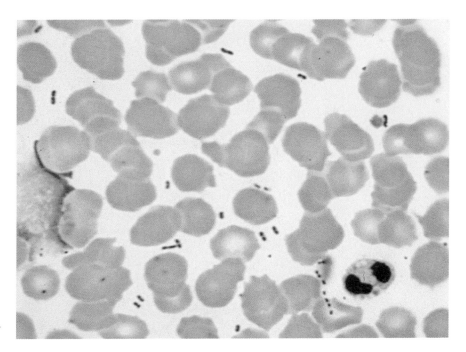

Figure IA2-28

Cell Type

Neutrophil, monocyte

Description

Microorganisms in cytoplasm

Clinical Conditions

■ Microbial infections

Toxic Granulation

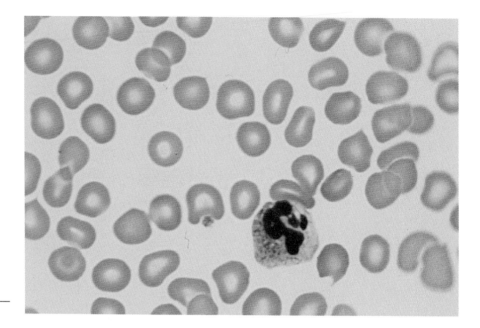

Figure IA2-29

Cell Type

Neutrophil

Description

Heavy, coarse, dark-blue primary cytoplasmic granules
Strong peroxidase reactivity

Clinical Conditions

- Infections
- Burns
- Drug intoxication
- Inflammation
- Growth factor therapy

Vacuolization

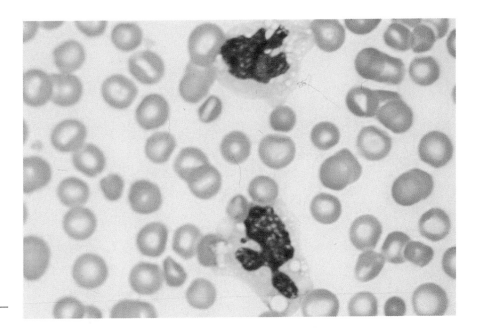

Figure **IA2-30**

Cell Type

Neutrophil, monocyte

Description

Vacuoles (holes) in cytoplasm

Clinical Conditions

- Severe infection
- Cell degeneration
- Phagocytosis
- Burns
- Toxins

LE Cell

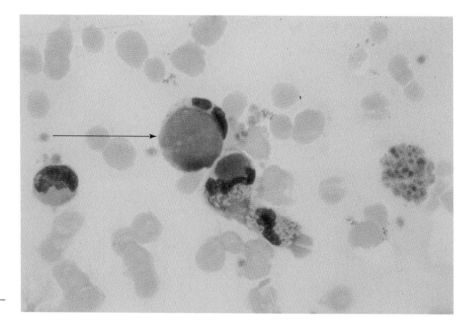

Figure IA2-31

Cell Type

Neutrophil

Description

Large, spherical body in cytoplasm is homogeneous, has no nuclear structure, and
stains pale purple; nucleus of cell is pushed to periphery and appears to wrap
around cytoplasmic inclusion

Clinical Conditions

■ Systemic lupus erythematosus

MALIGNANT GRANULOCYTES

Type I Myeloblast

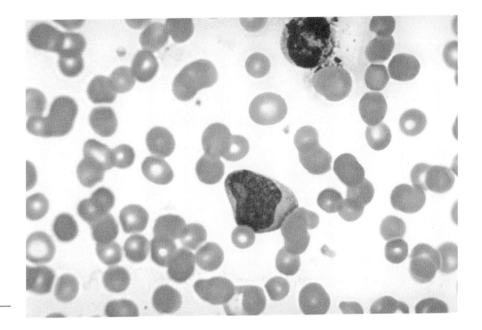

Figure **IA2-32**

Size: 10–18 μ

Nucleus

Shape: Oval or round
N/C Ratio: 6:1–7:1
Color: Dark purple
Chromatin: Fine
Nucleoli: 1–3

Cytoplasm

Color: Light to medium blue
Contents: Without azurophilic granules

Clinical Conditions

- Acute myelocytic leukemia minimally differentiated (M0)
- Acute myelocytic leukemia without maturation (M1)
- Acute myelocytic leukemia with maturation (M2)
- Acute myelomonocytic leukemia (M4)
- Erythroleukemia (M6a)
- Myeloproliferative diseases—CML, CIMF

Type II Myeloblast

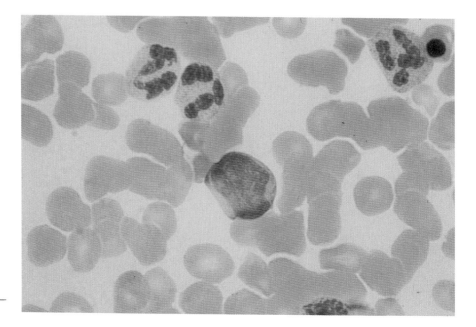

Figure IA2-33

Size: 10–18 μ

Nucleus

Shape: Oval or round
N/C Ratio: Slightly lower than a type I
Color: Dark purple
Chromatin: Slightly more condensed than a type I
Nucleoli: 2–5

Cytoplasm

Color: Medium blue
Contents: <20 azurophilic granules and may have Auer rods

Clinical Conditions

■ Acute myelocytic leukemia without maturation (M1)
■ Acute myelocytic leukemia with maturation (M2)
■ Acute myelomonocytic leukemia (M4)
■ Erythroleukemia (M6a)
■ Myeloproliferative diseases—CML, CIMF

Type III Myeloblast

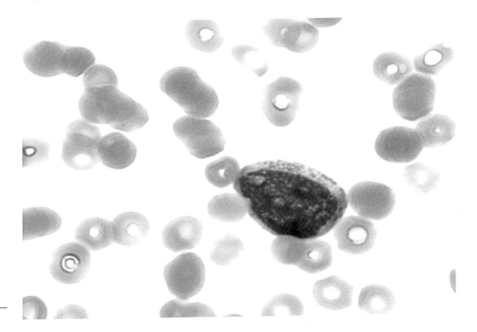

Figure IA2-34

Size: 10–18 μ

Nucleus

Shape: Oval or round
N/C Ratio: Lower than a type I
Location: Centrally located
Color: Dark purple
Chromatin: Slightly more condensed than type II
Nucleoli: Less visible

Cytoplasm

Color: Medium blue
Contents: >20 azurophilic granules but do not obscure the nucleus

Clinical Conditions

■ Acute myelocytic leukemia with maturation (M2)

Abnormal Promyelocyte

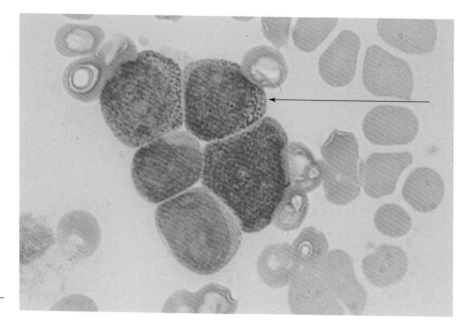

Figure IA2-35

Size: 18–25 μ

Nucleus

Shape: Round or, more commonly, reniform or bilobed
N/C Ratio: 2:1
Color: Purple
Chromatin: Relatively fine, becoming coarser
Nucleoli: 2–3, varying from visible to indistinct

Cytoplasm

Hypergranular Type:

Color: Intensely basophilic
Contents: Large red to purple granules; Auer rods may be numerous and intertwined, giving a haystack appearance (faggot cells); may obscure the nucleus

Microgranular Type:

Color: Moderately basophilic
Contents: Small, indistinct granules that are difficult to see with the light microscope; Auer rods are often found but not as abundant as those found in the hypergranular type

Clinical Condition

■ Acute promyelocytic leukemia (M3, M3v)

ABNORMAL MATURATION

Dysgranulopoiesis

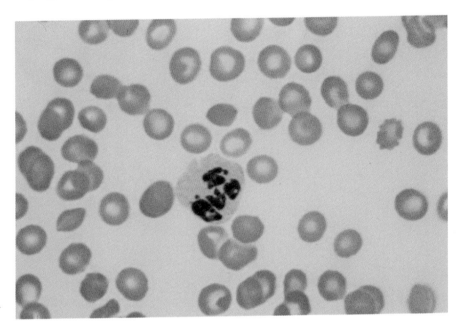

Figure IA2-36

Cell Type

Granulocyte cell line

Description

Nuclear/cytoplasmic asynchrony
Cytoplasm shows persistence of basophilia and may exhibit enlarged granules, hypogranulation, or agranularity
Nuclear asynchrony includes hypersegmentation or hyposegmentation

Clinical Conditions

■ Myelodysplastic syndromes
■ Some leukemias

Giant Myelocytes, Metamyelocytes, and Bands

Metamyelocyte ——→

Band ——→

Myelocyte ——→

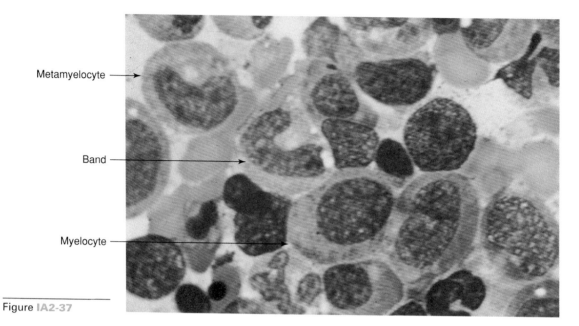

Figure IA2-37

Cell Type

Myelocyte, metamyelocyte, band

Description

Giant myelocytes are 17–26 μ; nucleus is round, oval, or flattened on one side, dark purple, coarse chromatin, and no visible nucleoli; cytoplasm is pinkish-blue with variable numbers of granules

Giant metamyelocytes are 15–22 μ; typical dark purple, kidney-shaped nucleus; cytoplasm is pink-blue with pinkish to reddish-blue granules

Giant bands are 14–20 μ; dark purple nucleus is band shaped; cytoplasm is pink-blue with pinkish-blue granules

Clinical Conditions

■ Folate deficiency
■ Vitamin B_{12} deficiency
■ Chemotherapy (folate antagonists)

MONOCYTES

Monocyte Maturation Series

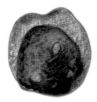

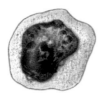

Figure **IA2-38**

Monoblast

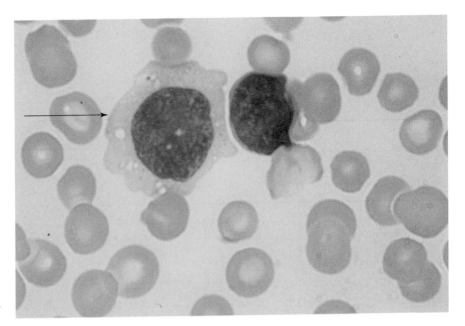

Figure IA2-39

Size: 14–20 μ

Nucleus

Shape: Round or oval
N/C Ratio: 3:1–1:1
Color: Light bluish-purple
Chromatin: Fine and distinct
Nucleoli: 1–5

Cytoplasm

Color: Blue-gray
Contents: No granules

Clinical Conditions

- Acute myelomonocytic leukemia (M4)
- Acute monoblastic leukemia (M5a)
- Acute monocytic leukemia (M5b)

Promonocyte

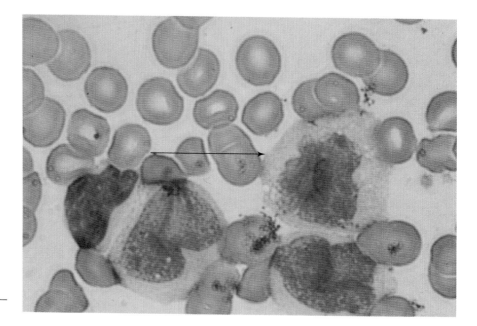

Figure IA2-40

Size: 14–20 μ

Nucleus

Shape: Oval or indented
N/C Ratio: 2:1–1:1
Color: Light bluish–purple
Chromatin: Fine reticular pattern
Nucleoli: 1–5

Cytoplasm

Color: Blue-gray, finely granular (ground glass) appearance
Contents: Many fine, dustlike, bluish granules; occasional vacuole

Clinical Conditions

- Acute myelomonocytic leukemia (M4)
- Acute monoblastic leukemia (M5a)
- Acute monocytic leukemia (M5b)
- Myelodysplastic/myeloproliferative diseases—chronic myelomonocytic leukemia (CMML)

Monocyte

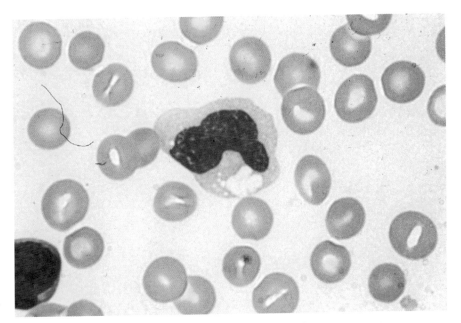

Figure IA2-41

Size: 14–21 μ

Nucleus

Shape: Horseshoe shaped or indented; nuclear folding may give the appearance of brainlike convolutions
N/C Ratio: 1:1
Color: Dark purple
Chromatin: Fine, delicate strands in linear arrangement with light spaces between strands
Nucleoli: None

Cytoplasm

Color: Blue-gray, finely granular (ground glass) appearance
Contents: Many fine, dustlike, bluish granules; occasional vacuole and blunt pseudopods

Clinical Conditions

■ Myelodysplastic/myeloproliferative diseases—CMML, juvenile myelomonocytic leukemia (JMML)
■ Myeloproliferative diseases—CML (few cases)
■ Severe infections

LYMPHOCYTES

Lymphocyte Maturation Series

Figure IA2-42

Lymphoblast

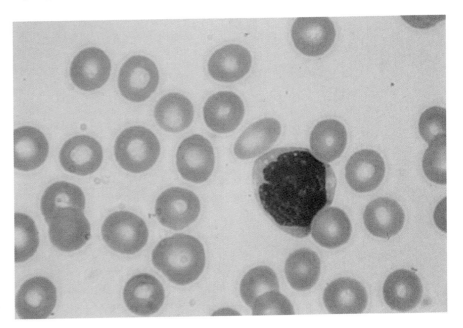

Figure IA2-43

Size: 10–22 μ

Nucleus

Shape: Round or oval, centrally or eccentrically placed
N/C Ratio: 7:1–4:1
Color: Reddish-purple
Chromatin: Fine, lacy pattern to moderately coarse
Nucleoli: 1–2 prominent

Cytoplasm

Color: Moderate to dark blue
Contents: Smooth, no granules, occasional vacuoles

Clinical Conditions

■ Precursor lymphoblastic leukemia (L_1, L_2)
■ Burkitt lymphoma (L_3)
■ Lymphoblastic lymphoma

Mature Lymphocyte

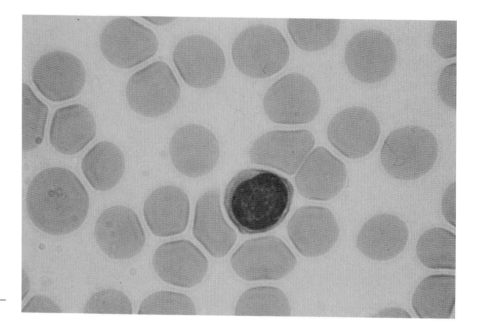

Size: 7–15 μ

Nucleus

Shape: Round or slightly indented, eccentric
N/C Ratio: 3:1
Color: Deep purple–blue
Chromatin: Course and clumped
Nucleoli: None visible

Cytoplasm

Color: Sky blue to deep blue
Contents: Scant and usually nongranular; few azurophilic granules may be seen

REACTIVE LYMPHOCYTES

Reactive Lymphocytes (Atypical Lymphocytes)

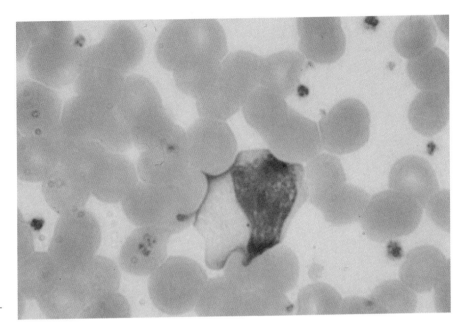

Figure IA2-45

Cell Type

Lymphocyte

Description

Cell size ranges from 10–25 μ

Nucleus can be oval, notched, indented, or elongated

One or more large nucleoli may be visible

Cytoplasm is often abundant and stains pale to deep blue and darker at periphery; may be partially indented by adjacent red cells; few lavender granules and/or vacuoles

Clinical Conditions

■ Infectious mononucleosis

■ Other viral diseases including cytomegalovirus, toxoplasmosis, hepatitis, and cat scratch fever

Cleaved Cell (Butt Cell)

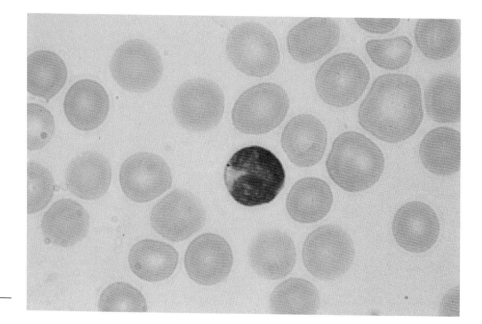

Figure IA2-46

Cell Type

Lymphocyte

Description

Small, mature lymphocyte with cleaved nucleus

Clinical Conditions

- Pertussis (Whooping cough)
- Lymphoma
- Chronic lymphocytic leukemia

Immunoblast

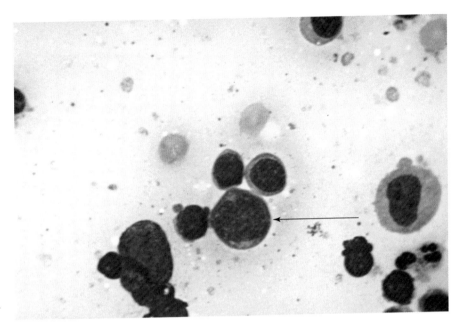

Figure **IA2-47**

Cell Type

Lymphocyte

Description

Large cell (12–25 μ) with bluish-purple nucleus and fine chromatin pattern with
  several prominent nucleoli
Cytoplasm is deep blue

Clinical Conditions

■ Viral and nonviral infections
■ Immune disorders

Large Granular Lymphocyte

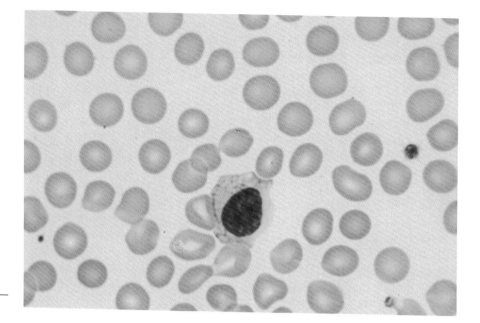

Cell Type

Lymphocyte

Description

Large cells (14–16 μ) with moderate to abundant pale blue cytoplasm
Prominent azurophilic granules

Clinical Conditions

- T-gamma lymphoproliferative disease
- Large granular lymphocytic leukemia
- NK cell leukemia

Large Lymphocyte

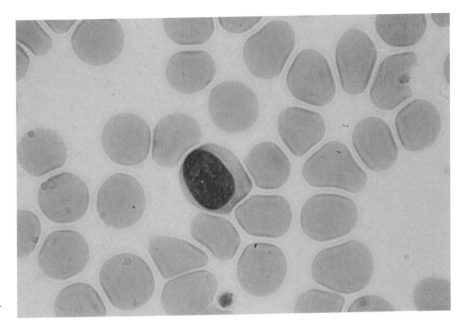

Cell Type

Lymphocyte

Description

Nucleus is round or oval, may be slightly indented, with coarse chromatin pattern and no visible nucleoli; moderate, pale-blue cytoplasm with rare purplish-red granules

Clinical Conditions

■ 10–12% of lymphocytes is normal

Plasmacytoid Lymphocyte

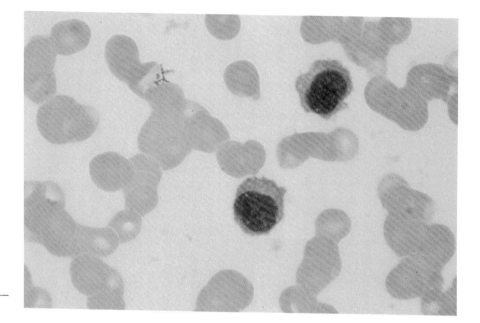

Figure IA2-50

Cell Type

Lymphocyte

Description

Cell is intermediated between small lymphocyte and plasma cell (9–20 μ); nucleus is centrally to slightly eccentrically located, indented or oval, with a developing perinuclear halo; chromatin strands are heavy or in dense blocks; cytoplasm is intensely basophilic and may contain few vacuoles

Clinical Conditions

- Viral and nonviral infections
- Immune disorders
- Plasma cell myeloma
- Waldenström macroglobulinemia

MALIGNANT LYMPHOCYTES

Chronic Lymphocytic Leukemia Lymphocyte

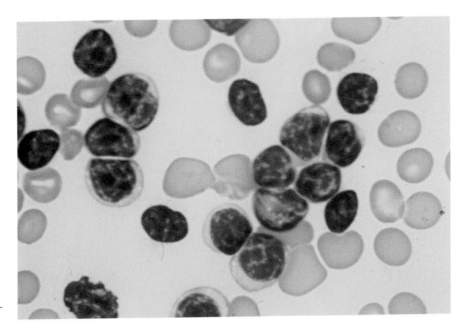

Figure **IA2-51**

Cell Type

Lymphocyte

Description

Cell size ranges from 10–15 μ
Nucleus is round, with an N/C ratio of 7:1–3:1
Chromatin is clumped and may show a compartmentalization phenomenon
Nucleoli are inconspicuous or not visible
Cytoplasm is sparse to abundant, clear, and lightly basophilic

Clinical Conditions

■ Chronic lymphocytic leukemia
■ Prolymphocytic leukemia/chronic lymphocytic leukemia
■ Prolymphocytic leukemia

Hairy Cell

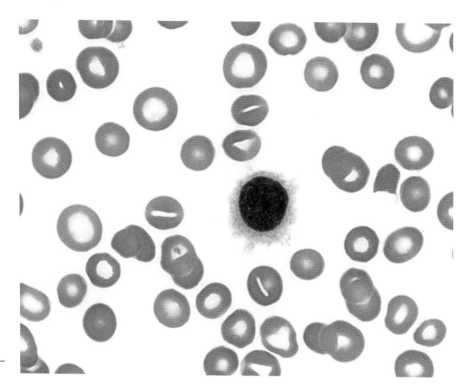

Cell Type

Lymphocyte

Description

Scant to abundant agranular, light grayish–blue cytoplasm; numerous, irregular
   cytoplasmic projections give a hairlike or ruffled appearance to plasma
   membrane; nucleus is round or oval and may occasionally appear kidney or
   hourglass shaped; loose and lacy chromatin pattern with one or two visible
   nucleoli

Clinical Condition

■ Hairy cell leukemia

L₁ Lymphoblast

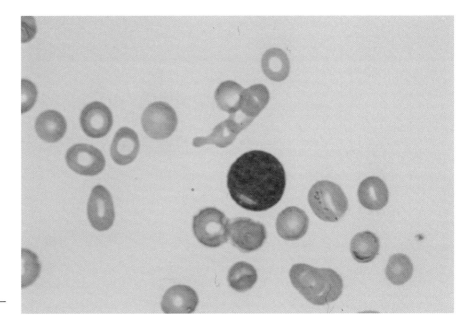

Figure IA2-53

Cell Type

Lymphoblast

Description

Cell size ranges from 10–14 μ
Nuclear shape is regular or small cleaved and indented
Purple nucleus has a homogeneous and condensed chromatin pattern
Nucleoli are inconspicuous or not visible (0-1)
Scanty cytoplasm is moderately basophilic and rarely vacuolated

Clinical Condition

■ Precursor lymphoblastic leukemia

L₂ Lymphoblast

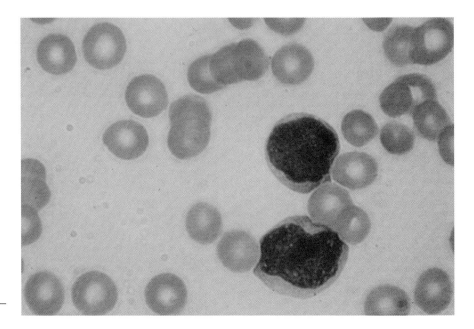

Figure IA2-54

Cell Type

Lymphoblast

Description

Cell size ranges from 14–22 μ
Nucleus has an irregular or indented shape
N/C ratio is average (4:1)
Nucleus is purplish-red, with variable heterogeneous chromatin
One to two nucleoli are often prominent
Cytoplasm is variable but occasionally intensely basophilic and rarely vacuolated

Clinical Condition

■ Precursor lymphoblastic leukemia

L₃ Lymphoblast

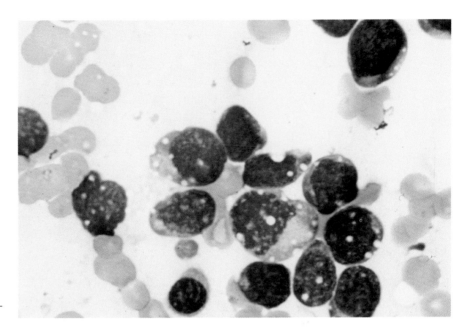

Cell Type

Lymphoblast

Description

Cell size ranges from 14–18 μ

Nucleus is oval to round, purple, and has a finely stippled and homogeneous chromatin pattern

N/C ratio is 5:1–4:1

One to two nucleoli are often prominent

Cytoplasm is intensely basophilic with prominent vacuolization

Clinical Condition

■ Burkitt lymphoma

■ Acute lymphoblastic leukemia (L3)

Prolymphocyte

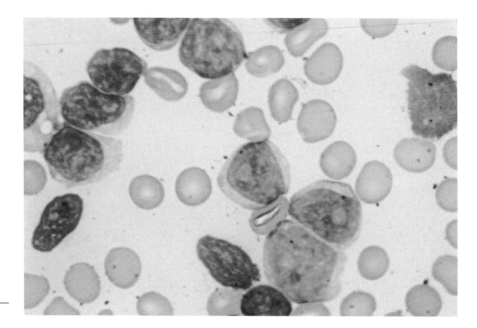

Cell Type

Lymphocyte

Size: 10–15 μ

Description

Round, centrally placed nucleus that is reddish-purple, with coarse, clumped
   chromatin
N/C ratio is 3:1–4:1
One prominent nucleolus
Cytoplasm is abundant; light to moderate blue

Clinical Conditions

■ Chronic lymphocytic leukemia (<11% prolymphocytes)
■ Prolymphocytic leukemia (>55% prolymphocytes)
■ Chronic lymphocytic leukemia/prolymphocytic leukemia (11–55%
   prolymphocytes)

LYMPHOMA CELLS

Lymphoblastic Lymphoma Cell

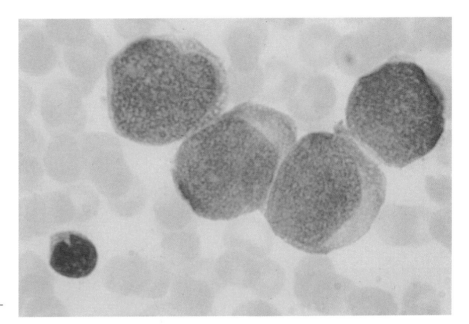

Figure IA2-57

Cell Type

Lymphoblast

Description

Cell size is variable
Nucleus is indented or convoluted, with fine chromatin pattern and small,
   inconspicuous nucleoli
Cytoplasm is scant

Clinical Condition

■ Lymphoblastic lymphoma

Reed-Sternberg Cell

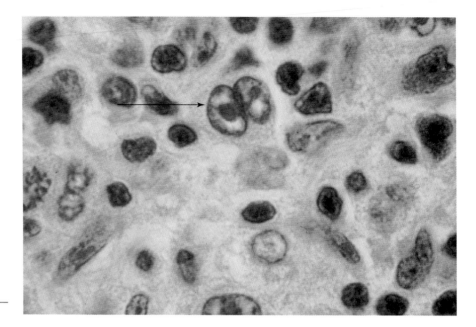

Figure IA2-58

Cell Type

Lymphocytic lineage

Description

A large cell (50–100 μ) with an abundance of cytoplasm
Nucleus is often bilobed or binucleated, with prominent large nucleoli resembling
   owl eyes; the two halves of a binucleated cell often appear as mirror images
Not found in peripheral blood; found in lymph nodes

Clinical Condition

■ Hodgkin lymphoma

Sézary Cell

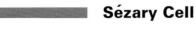

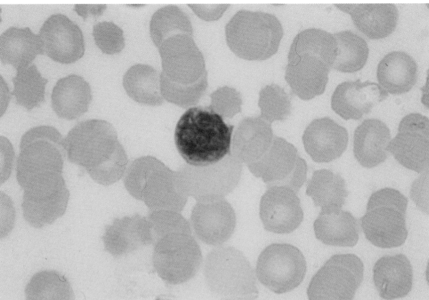

Figure IA2-59

Cell Type

Lymphocyte

Description

Small and large cell ranging from 8–30 μ

Nucleus has brainlike convolutions and is dark purple, with moderately coarse chromatin; nucleoli are not visible

Cytoplasm is scanty and pale to deep blue with occasional vacuoles

Clinical Conditions

■ Cutaneous T-cell lymphoma (mycosis fungoides, Sézary syndrome)
■ T_4 lymphomas involving the skin

Small Cleaved Lymphoma Cell

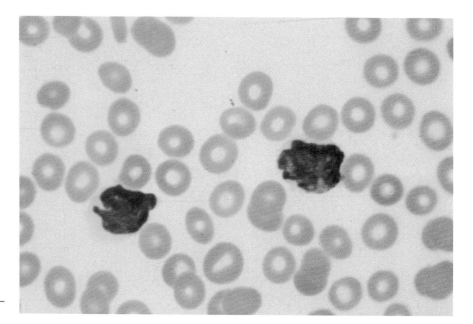

Figure IA2-60

Cell Type

Lymphoma cell

Description

Cell size is 6–12 μ; nucleus is twisted, angulated, and indented, with clumped
   chromatin and no nucleoli
Cytoplasm is scant to imperceptible

Clinical Condition

■ Small cleaved cell lymphoma

Small B Lymphoma Cell

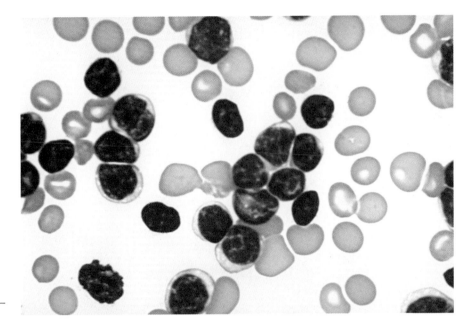

Figure **IA2-61**

Cell Type

Lymphocyte

Description

Cell is 10–25 μ; round nucleus has clumped chromatin and may show a
  compartmentalization phenomenon
Nucleoli are inconspicuous or not visible
Cytoplasm is sparse to abundant and clear and lightly basophilic

Clinical Condition

■ Lymphoma

PLASMACYTES

Plasma Cell Series

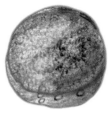

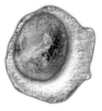

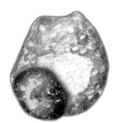

Figure IA2-62

Plasmablast

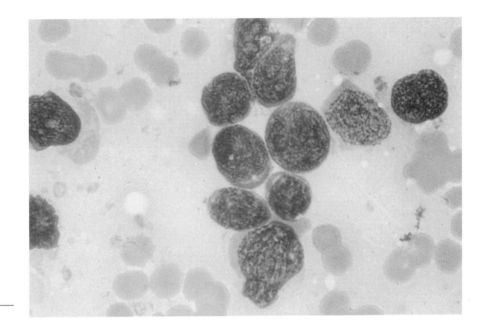

Figure IA2-63

Size: 12–15 μ

Nucleus

Shape: Round
N/C Ratio: 5:1–4:1
Color: Purplish-red
Chromatin: Fine and linear strands
Nucleoli: 1–2

Cytoplasm

Color: Blue
Contents: Nongranular

Clinical Conditions

■ Plasma cell leukemia
■ Plasma cell myeloma

Proplasmacyte

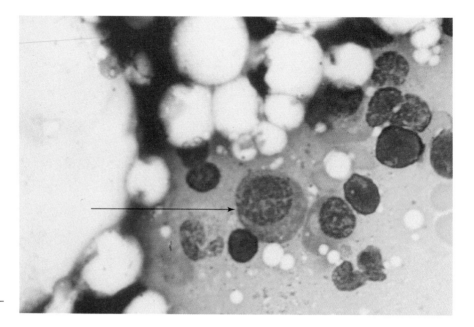

Figure IA2-64

Size: 12–15 μ

Nucleus

Shape: Round, eccentrically placed
N/C Ratio: 5:1–4:1
Color: Purplish-red
Chromatin: Moderately clumped
Nucleoli: 0–2

Cytoplasm

Color: Dark blue, prominent light area next to nucleus
Contents: Nongranular

Clinical Conditions

- Plasma cell leukemia
- Plasma cell myeloma
- Waldenström macroglobulinemia
- Response to infection

Plasma Cell

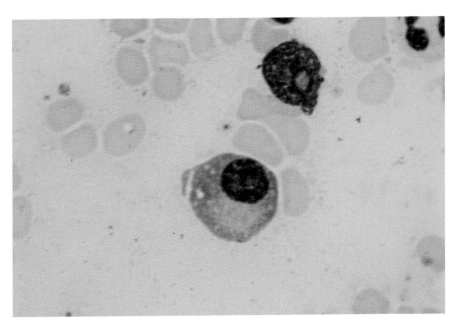

Figure **IA2-65**

Cell Type

Plasma cell

Description

Size ranges from 9–20 μ
Dark purple nucleus is ovoid and eccentrically placed, with a wheel-spoke pattern
No nucleoli
Cytoplasm is abundant and deep blue with a clear area next to the nucleus

Clinical Conditions

■ Plasma cell dyscrasias
■ Response to infections

ABNORMAL PLASMA CELLS AND INCLUSIONS

Bilobed Plasma Cell

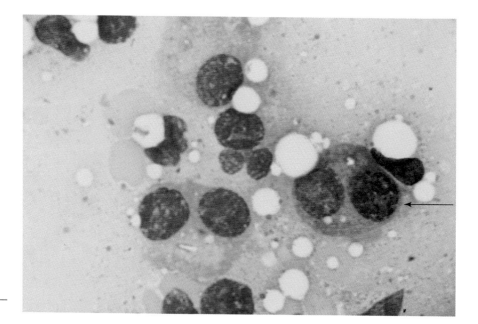

Figure IA2-66

Cell Type

Plasma cell

Description

Dark purple nucleus is bilobed rather than ovoid
Cytoplasm is pale to deeply basophilic

Clinical Condition

■ Plasma cell dyscrasias

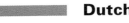

Dutcher Body

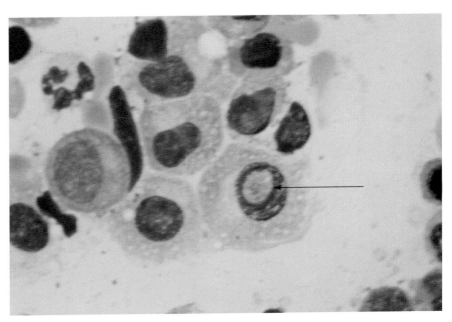

Figure **IA2-67**

Cell Type

Plasma cell

Description

Intranuclear protein inclusions resulting from membrane-bound cytoplasm in the nucleus

Clinical Condition

■ Plasma cell dyscrasias

Flaming Plasma Cell

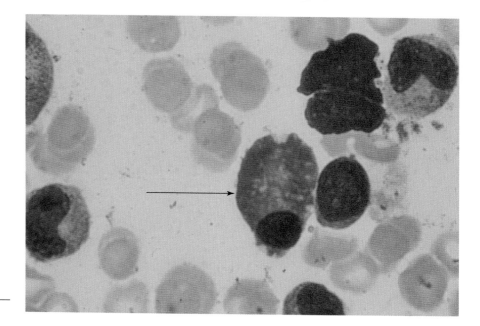

Cell Type

Plasma cell

Description

Cytoplasmic immunoglobulin (often IgA) accumulating in the peripheral
cytoplasm; stains reddish-purple

Clinical Condition

■ Plasma cell dyscrasias

Mott Cell (Grape Cell)

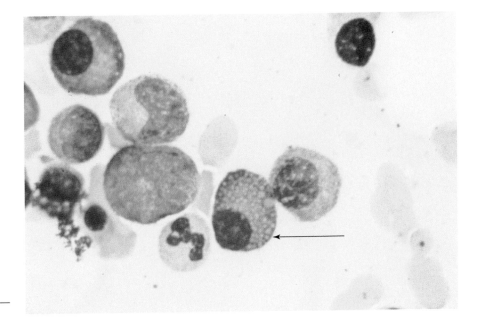

Cell Type

Plasma cell

Description

Cytoplasm filled with Russell bodies resembling clusters of grapes

Clinical Condition

■ Plasma cell dyscrasias

Russell Bodies

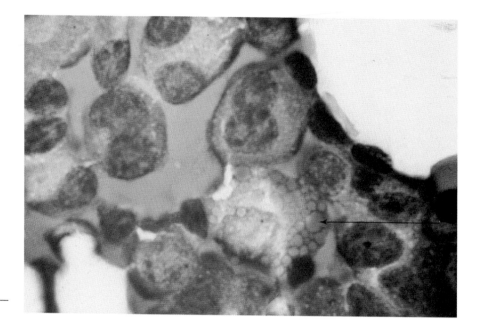

Cell Type

Plasma cell

Description

Individual globules of immunoglobulin in cytoplasm, which represent rough endoplasmic reticulum, smooth endoplasmic reticulum, and Golgi filled with immunoglobulin due to secretory obstruction; globules stain pink or blue depending on pH; if immunoglobulin disappears, colorless vacuoles result

Clinical Condition

■ Plasma cell dyscrasias

CHAPTER

3

Megakaryocytes

NORMAL MEGAKARYOCYTIC MATURATION SERIES

Normal Megakaryocytic Series

Figure IA3-1

Megakaryoblast

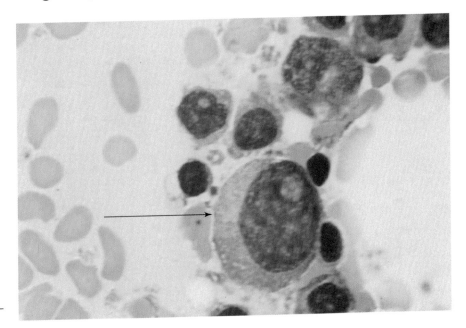

Figure IA3-2

Size: 20–50 μ

Nucleus

Shape: Round, oval, or kidney shaped
N/C Ratio: 5:1–3:1
Color: Reddish-purple to purple
Chromatin: Fine, distinct strands to dense chromatin
Nucleoli: Several, often indistinct or maybe more distinct in larger blasts

Cytoplasm

Color: Moderate to dark blue
Contents: Blunt cytoplasmic extensions; no granules to fine azurophilic granules in the larger blasts

Clinical Conditions

■ Acute megakaryoblastic leukemia (M7)
■ Myeloproliferative diseases—CML, CIMF
■ Myelodysplastic syndromes

Promegakaryocyte

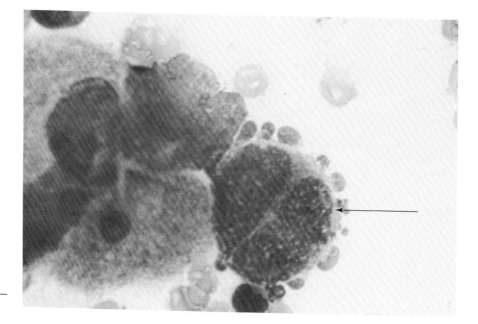

Size: 20–80 μ

Nucleus

Shape: Irregularly indented, with 2–4 lobes
N/C Ratio: 1:1
Color: Dark purple
Chromatin: Fine; condensed near periphery
Nucleoli: Several

Cytoplasm

Color: Moderate blue to pinkish-blue
Contents: Few bluish granules; development of demarcation membrane system forming small cytoplasmic extensions

Clinical Conditions

- Acute megakaryoblastic leukemia (M7)
- Myeloproliferative diseases—CML, CIMF, essential thrombocytopenia (ET)
- Myelodysplastic syndromes
- Acute myelocytic leukemia with multilineage dysplasia

Megakaryocyte

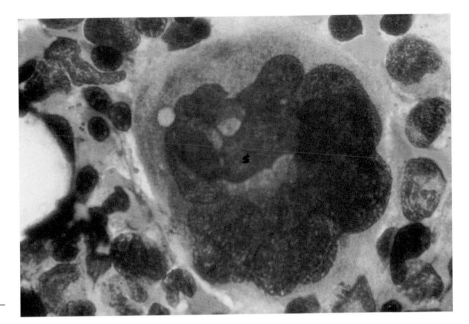

Figure IA3-4

Size: 40–100 μ

Nucleus

Shape: Multilobular
N/C Ratio: 1:1–1:12
Color: Dark purple
Chromatin: Coarse, linear
Nucleoli: None

Cytoplasm

Color: Pinkish-blue
Contents: Numerous reddish-blue granules

Clinical Conditions

- Acute megakaryoblastic leukemia (M7)
- Myeloproliferative diseases—CML, CIMF
- Myelodysplastic syndromes
- Acute myelocytic leukemia with multilineage dysplasia

Platelets

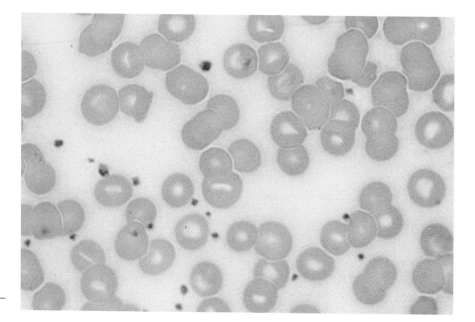

Size: 1–4 μ

Nucleus

None

Cytoplasm

Color: Light blue
Contents: Small reddish-blue granules

Clinical Conditions

- Acute megakaryoblastic leukemia (M7)
- Myelodysplastic syndromes—RAEB, 5q- syndrome
- Myelodysplastic/myeloproliferative diseases—CMML
- Myeloproliferative diseases—CML, polycythemia vera (PV), ET, CIMF
- Idiopathic thrombocytopenic purpura
- Microangiopathic hemolytic anemias—hemolytic uremic syndrome (HUS), disseminated intravascular coagulation (DIC), thrombocytopenic purpura (TTP)

ABNORMAL MEGAKARYOCYTIC CELLS

Giant Platelet

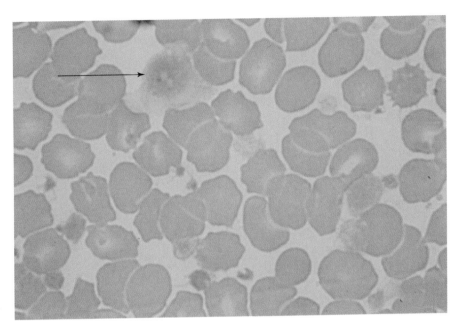

Figure **IA3-6**

Cell Type

Platelet

Description

Platelet as large as or larger than erythrocytes or granulocytes; light blue with small reddish-blue granules or degranulated (pale blue with no granules)

Clinical Conditions

■ May-Hegglin syndrome
■ Myelofibrosis
■ Thrombasthenia
■ Myeloproliferative diseases
■ Splenectomy
■ Myelodysplastic syndromes

Large Megakaryocyte

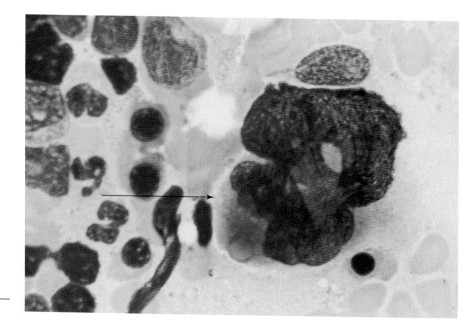

Figure IA3-7

Cell Type

Megakaryocyte

Description

Large megakaryocyte with hyperlobulation

Clinical Conditions

■ Vitamin B_{12} deficiency
■ Folic acid deficiency
■ Myelodysplastic syndromes
■ Idiopathic thrombocytopenic purpura

Large Mononuclear Megakaryocyte

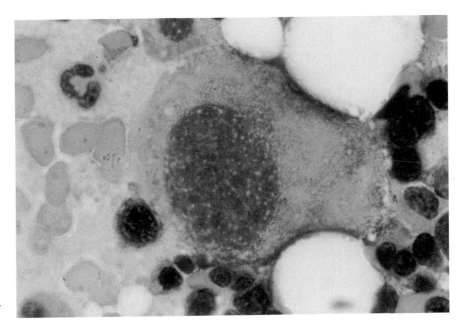

Figure IA3-8

Cell Type

Megakaryocyte

Description

Large megakaryocyte with a single nucleus

Clinical Conditions

- Myelodysplastic syndromes
- Acute megakaryoblastic leukemia (M7)

Micromegakaryocyte

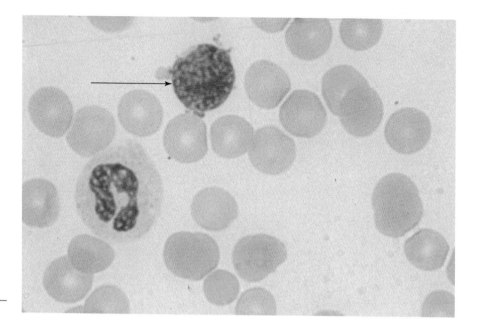

Figure IA3-9

Cell Type

Megakaryocyte

Description

Small megakaryocyte about the size of a lymphocyte
Single-lobed nucleus resembles medium-sized lymphocyte
One or more platelet fragments attached to nucleus or scant cytoplasm

Clinical Conditions

■ Myeloproliferative diseases
■ Myelodysplastic syndromes
■ Acute megakaryoblastic leukemia (M7)

Vacuolated Megakaryocyte

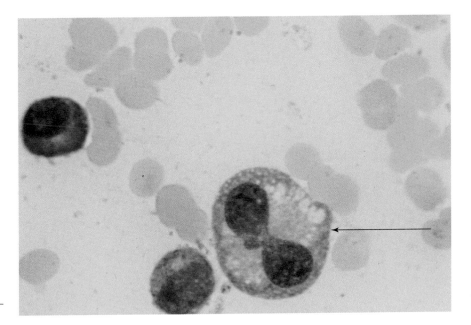

Figure IA3-10

Cell Type

Megakaryocyte

Description

Megakaryocyte or promegakaryocyte with a single or bilobed nucleus
Vacuoles in the basophilic or minimal granule-forming cytoplasm

Clinical Conditions

■ Myelodysplastic syndromes
■ Acute megakaryoblastic leukemia (M7)

CHAPTER 4

Comparison of Cells

Myeloblast, Myelocyte

Myelocyte ——————————————→

Myeloblast ——————————————→

Myeloblast

Fine nuclear chromatin
Moderate amount of agranular blue cytoplasm
N/C ratio higher

Myelocyte

Moderately clumped deep purple nucleus
Presence of some residual primary granules and the beginning of some secondary
   granule formation in the cytoplasm

Myeloblast, Promyelocyte, Myelocyte

Promyelocyte ————→

Myelocyte ————→

Myeloblast ————→

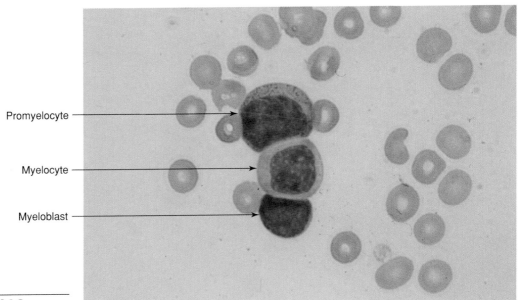

Figure IA4-2

Myeloblast

Highest N/C ratio
Finest nuclear chromatin pattern

Promyelocyte

Presence of primary azurophilic granules
Cytoplasm is moderate blue color

Myelocyte

Lowest N/C ratio
Muddy gray cytoplasmic color
Secondary granules are present
Nuclear chromatin is more clumped

Myeloblast, Basophilic Normoblast

Myeloblast —

Basophilic
normoblast —

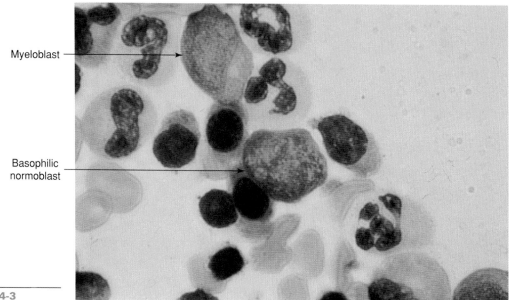

Figure IA4-3

Myeloblast

Finer nuclear chromatin pattern with visible nucleoli
Cytoplasm has a lighter blue color

Basophilic Normoblast

Nucleus has a more clumped chromatin pattern
Cytoplasm has a deeper blue color

Late Polychromatophilic Normoblast, Lymphocyte

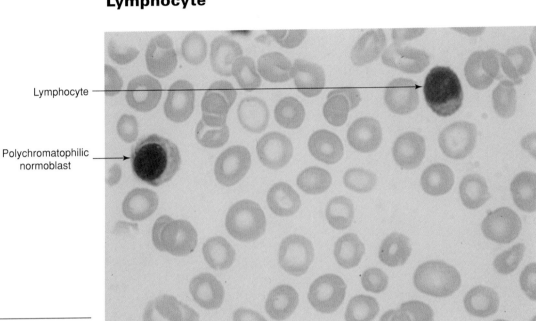

Lymphocyte

Polychromatophilic normoblast

Figure IA4-4

Late Polychromatophilic Normoblast

Nucleus is deep purple and slightly eccentric
Nuclear chromatin is intensely condensed
Cytoplasm is pink with a bluish tinge

Lymphocyte

Nucleus is pale purple and eccentric
Nuclear chromatin is moderately condensed
Cytoplasm is light blue and scanty

Monoblast, Promonocyte

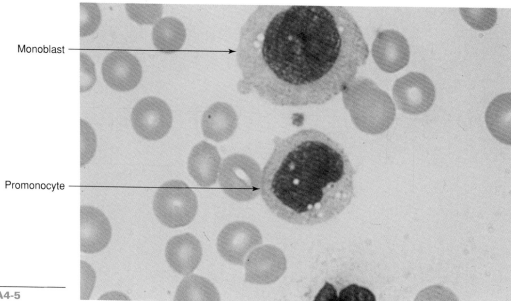

Monoblast —

Promonocyte —

Figure IA4-5

Monoblast

Larger cell
Round nucleus with cleave evident
One single nucleoli present
Similar cytoplasms

Promonocyte

Indented nucleus with a more condensed chromatin pattern

Monoblast, Myeloblast

Monoblast →

Myeloblast →

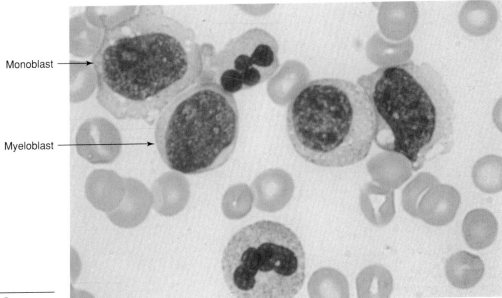

Figure IA4-6

Monoblast

More cytoplasm
Nucleus has finely dispersed chromatin with a vaguely noticeable cleave

Myeloblast

Higher N/C ratio
Finer chromatin pattern
Smaller cell

Monocyte, Reactive Lymphocyte

Reactive lymphocyte

Monocyte

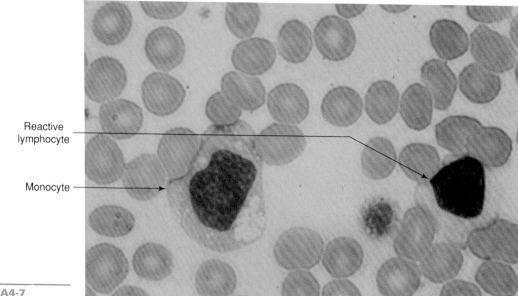

Figure IA4-7

Monocyte

Cell is larger
Lower N/C ratio
Finer nuclear chromatin pattern

Reactive Lymphocyte

Cell is smaller
Condensed nuclear chromatin pattern
Higher N/C ratio

Monocyte, Lymphocyte

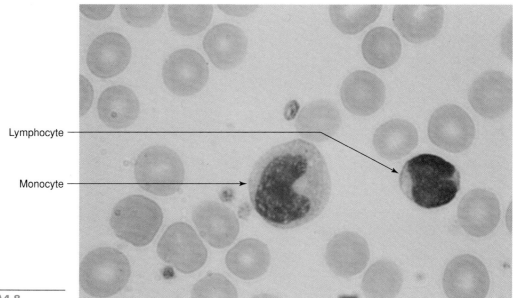

Lymphocyte

Monocyte

Figure **IA4-8**

Monocyte

Lower N/C ratio
Finer, lacy nuclear chromatin pattern
Nucleus is indented
Larger cell

Lymphocyte

Nucleus is indented
Intensely clumped nucleus
Higher N/C ratio

Pronormoblast, Myelocyte

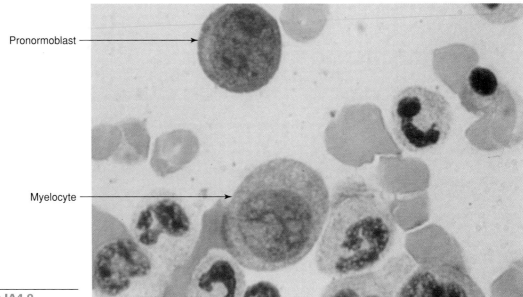

Pronormoblast ———————————→

Myelocyte ———————————→

Figure IA4-9

Pronormoblast

Nucleus is large, deep purple, and centrally located
Nuclear chromatin is finely stippled
Cytoplasm is intensely basophilic, with light areas of mitochondria
High N/C ratio

Myelocyte

Nucleus is light purple and slightly off center
Nuclear chromatin is moderately condensed, with a prominent nucleoli (nucleoli
   can still be present since this cell can still divide)
Cytoplasm is grayish-blue with a hint of pink granulation
Lower N/C ratio

Pronormoblast, Promyelocyte

Pronormoblast

Promyelocyte

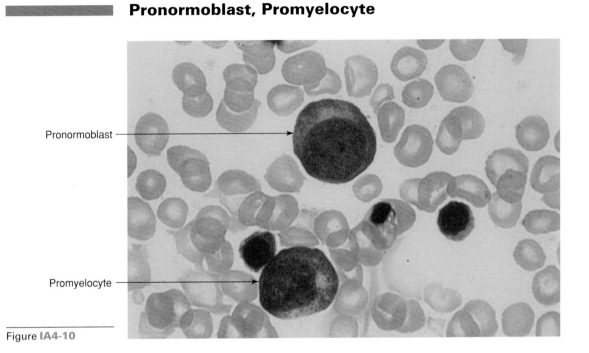

Figure IA4-10

Pronormoblast

Nucleus is large, deep purple, and centrally located
Nuclear chromatin is finely stippled
Cytoplasm is intensely basophilic light areas of mitochondria
Light area next to the nucleus is the Golgi

Promyelocyte

Nucleus is purple and eccentrically located
Nuclear chromatin is finely condensed
Cytoplasm has numerous dark, primary granules that have begun to obscure the
    nucleus

Early Myelocyte, Late Myelocyte

Late ——→

Early ——→

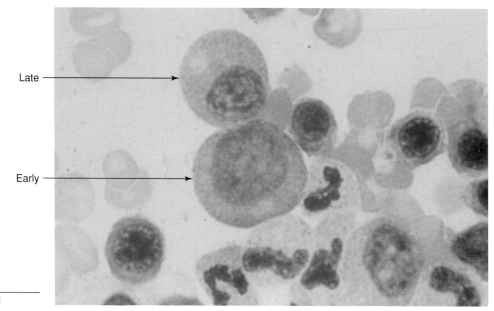

Early Myelocyte

Nucleus is light purple and slightly off center
Nuclear chromatin is moderately condensed, with a prominent nucleoli
Cytoplasm is grayish-blue, with a hint of pink granulation

Late Myelocyte

Nucleus is purple, oval, and eccentric
Nuclear chromatin is fairly clumped and has an aggregated pattern with no visible
nucleoli
Cytoplasm is granulated with pink secondary granules

Metamyelocyte, Neutrophilic Band, Neutrophil

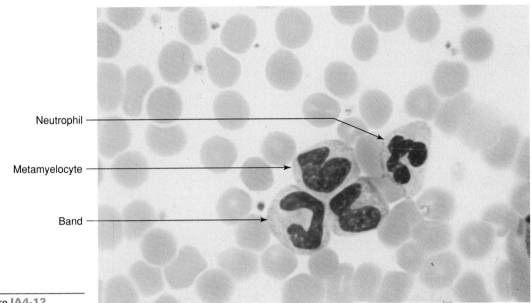

Neutrophil

Metamyelocyte

Band

Figure IA4-12

Metamyelocyte

Nucleus is deep purple and has a kidney to slightly indented shape
Nuclear chromatin is fairly coarse but not as clumped as the band or segmented
neutrophil

Neutrophilic Band

Nucleus is deep purple and markedly indented to make a band shape
Nuclear chromatin is intensely clumped

Segmented Neutrophil

Nucleus is deep purple and has a segmented shape
Nuclear chromatin is coarsely clumped
Cytoplasm for all three cells is basically the same and seldom helpful in
differentiating the cells

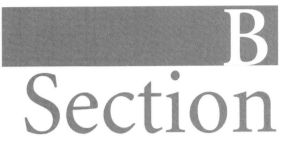

Section

Bone Marrow

CHAPTER

1

Cellularity

NORMAL CELLULARITY

Normal Adult Cellularity

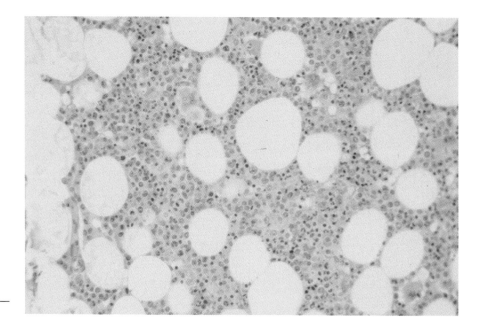

Figure **IB1-1**

Description

30–80% cellularity

Normal Elderly Cellularity

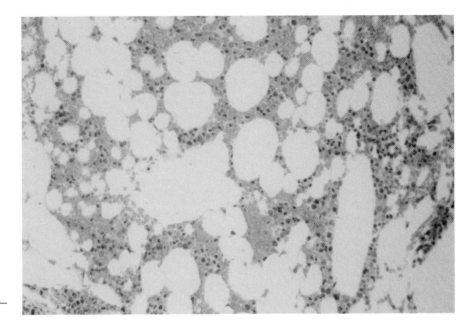

Figure IB1-2

Description

20–50% cellularity

Normal Adolescent Cellularity

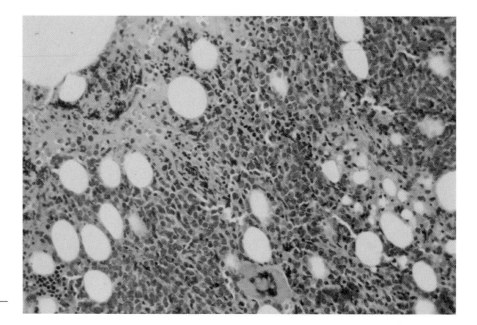

Figure IB1-3

Description

50–90% cellularity

Normal Newborn Cellularity

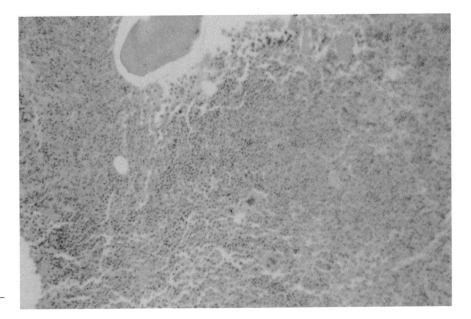

Figure IB1-4

Description

75–100% cellularity

Adult Hypocellularity

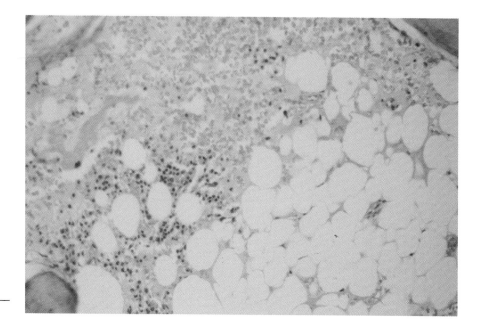

Figure **IB1-5**

Description

<20% cellularity

Clinical Conditions

■ Production disorder
■ Aplastic anemia
■ Anorexia nervosa

Adult Hypercellularity

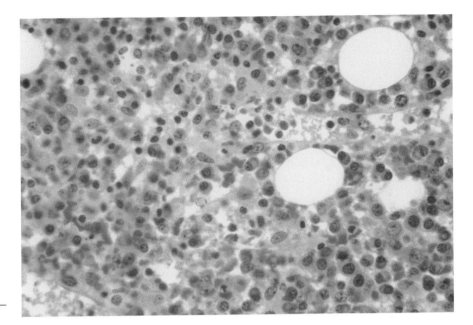

Description

>50% cellularity

Clinical Conditions

■ Ineffective hematopoiesis; increased peripheral destruction
■ Malignancies
■ Reactive processes

Erythropoiesis

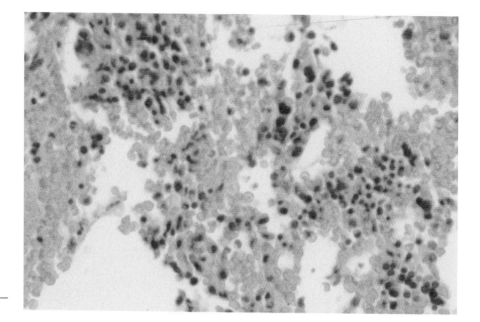

Description

>30% of marrow cellularity is erythrocytic

Clinical Conditions

- Increased M:E ratio—decreased production of erythrocytes
- Decreased M:E ratio—increased production of erythrocytes or ineffective erythropoiesis

Granulopoiesis

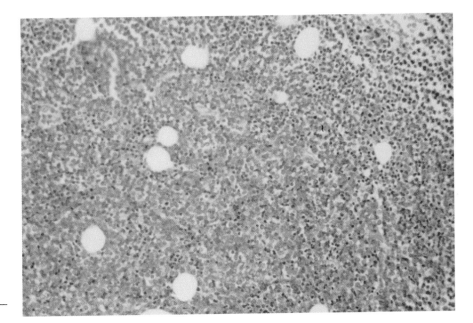

Figure IB1-8

Description

>40% of marrow cellularity represents granulopoiesis

Clinical Conditions

■ Increased M:E ratio—increased granulocyte production
■ Decreased M:E ratio—decreased granulocyte production

Lymphopoiesis

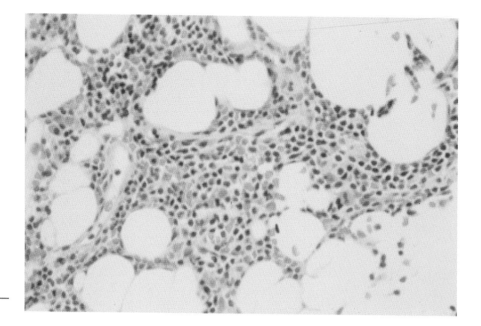

Description

>20% of marrow cellularity is lymphocytic cells

Clinical Conditions

- Lymphoproliferative disorders
- Plasmacytomas
- Marrow aplasias
- Chronic lymphocytic leukemia

Megakaryopoiesis

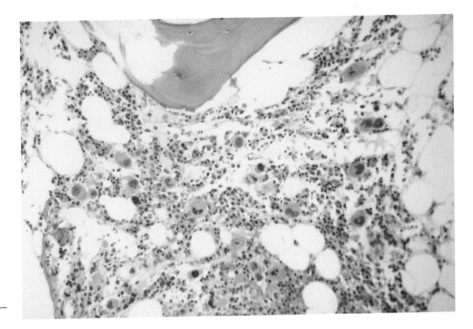

Figure **IB1-10**

Description

Usually see 1–5 megakaryocytes per 1000 cells

Clinical Conditions

- Idiopathic thrombocytopenic purpura
- Myeloproliferative syndromes
- Some myelodysplastic syndromes—5 q-syndrome
- Acute megakaryoblastic leukemia (M7)

CHAPTER

2

Cells of the Reticuloendothelial System

NORMAL CELLS

Macrophage

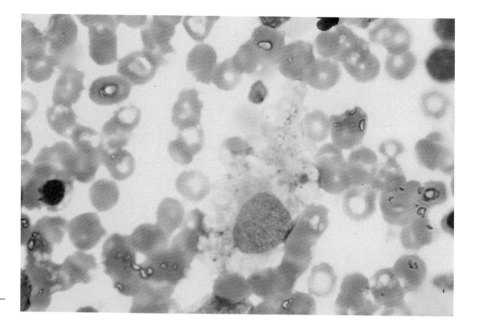

Figure **IB2-1**

Size: 15–80 μ

Nucleus

Shape: Egg-shaped, indented, elongated
N/C Ratio: 2:1–1:1
Color: Purple
Chromatin: Spongy
Nucleoli: None

Cytoplasm

Color: Sky blue
Contents: Coarse, azure granules; vacuoles; many neutral red bodies scattered
   throughout

Reticulum Cell

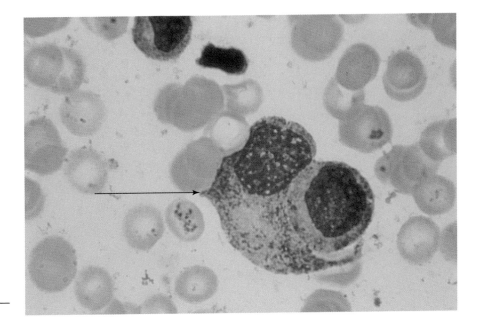

Figure IB2-2

Size: 20–30 μ

Nucleus

Shape: Round to oval
N/C Ratio: 1:1
Color: Purple with reddish hue
Chromatin: Fine, loosely bound but with areas of parachromatin
Nucleoli: 1 or more

Cytoplasm

Irregular outline
Color: Pale, blue, often retracted or folded, caused by smearing technique
Contents: Reticulin fibers that cause an azurophilic appearance; may contain
  phagocytized materials

ABNORMAL CELLS

Gaucher Cell

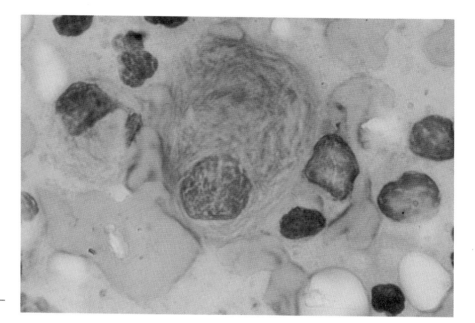

Figure IB2-3

Cell Type

Macrophage

Size: 20–80 μ

Description

A pale-staining cell; the cytoplasm is filled with a fibrillar lipid, which gives the appearance of crumpled tissue paper or a wrinkled look; the nucleus is small, round, and eccentrically placed

Clinical Conditions

- Gaucher disease
- Thalassemia (pseudo–Gaucher cells)
- Chronic myelocytic leukemia (pseudo–Gaucher cells)

Niemann-Pick Cell

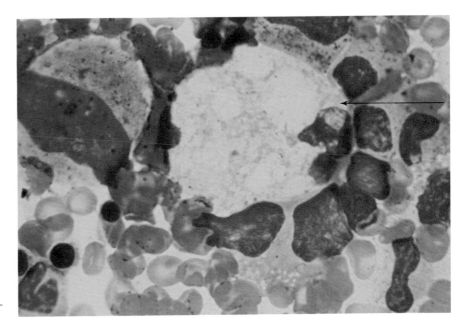

Figure **IB2-4**

Cell Type

Macrophage

Size: 20–90 μ

Cell Description

Pale staining; cytoplasm contains droplets of sphingomyelin, giving it a globular appearance; the nucleus is small, round, and eccentrically placed

Clinical Condition

■ Niemann-Pick disease

Sea-Blue Histiocyte

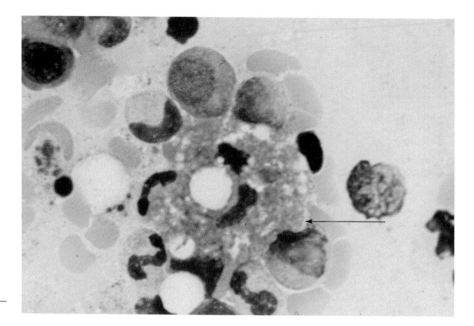

Figure IB2-5

Cell Type

Histiocyte

Size: 20–60 μ

Description

Cell containing granules that stain a sea-blue or blue-green; nucleus is small, round, and eccentric, with block chromatin

Clinical Conditions

- Sea-blue histiocytosis
- Pseudo–sea-blue histiocytes are seen in the following:
    - Thalassemia
    - Chronic myelocytic leukemia
    - Polycythemia vera
    - Sickle cell anemia
    - Sarcoidosis
    - Chronic granulomatous disease

CHAPTER

3

Nonhematopoietic Cells

Osteoblast

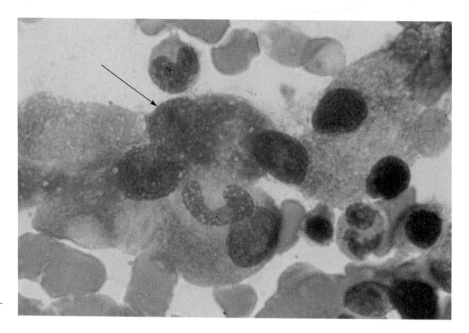

Figure IB3-1

Size: Frequently Found in Clumps, but Each Individual Cell Ranges from 25–50 μ

Nucleus

Shape: Oval or round; eccentric
N/C Ratio: 1:3–1:4
Color: Purple
Chromatin: Finely granular with clumps; some areas of parachromatin
Nucleoli: 1-3 present, small, light blue

Cytoplasm

Color: Pale blue to dark blue with blurred outlines
Contents: Round, pink-gray areas (archoplasm)

Osteoclast

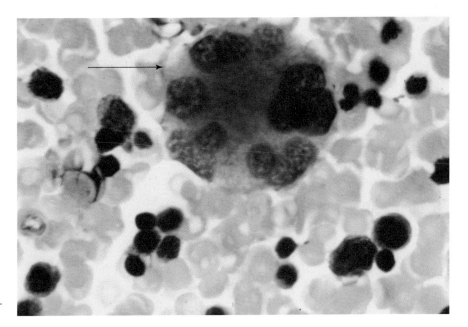

Figure IB3-2

Size: Usually > 100 μ

Nucleus

Polyploid and scattered throughout cell; not interconnected
Shape: Round
N/C Ratio: 4:1–2:1–1:1
Color: Purple
Chromatin: Dense
Nucleoli: Usually 1–2 present in each nucleus

Cytoplasm

Color: Light blue to pink, giving a cloudy appearance
Contents: Coarse granules

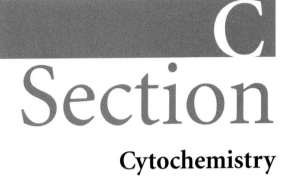

Section

Cytochemistry

CHAPTER

1

Cytochemical Stains

ACID PHOSPHATASE REACTION

With Tartrate Inhibition (TRAP)

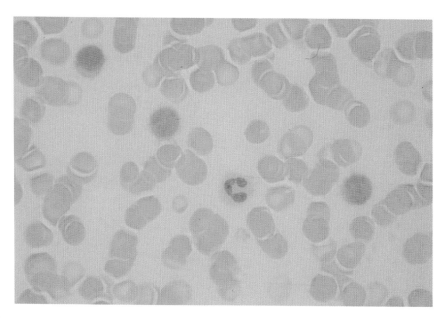

Figure **IC1-1**   Negative

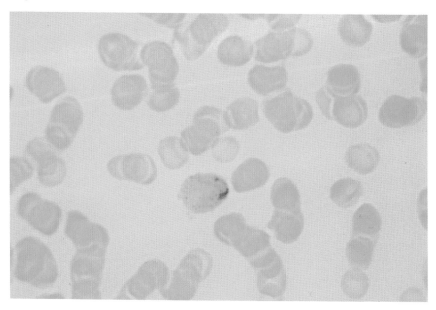

Figure **IC1-2**   Positive

Cell Type

Hairy cells, histiocytes, activated lymphocytes, and activated macrophages

Description

Acid phosphatase (isoenzyme 5) is resistant to tartrate
Hairy cells and histiocytes contain this acid phosphatase, are resistant to inhibition, and will demonstrate positivity (color is dependent on couplers used)

Clinical Conditions

- Hairy cell leukemia
- Gaucher disease

Without Tartrate Inhibition

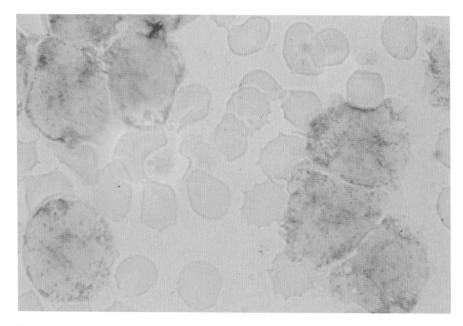

Positive

Cell Type

Most nucleated cells of the hematopoietic system and platelets

Description

Positivity is indicated by a diffuse granular red reaction product
The red product will disappear or contain only a small amount of reactivity after
    tartrate is added to the reaction
Focal positivity may be found in blasts of T-cell ALL

Clinical Conditions

- Some T-cell precursor lymphoblastic leukemia
- T-cell chronic lymphocytic leukemic
- T-cell prolymphocytic leukemia

NONSPECIFIC ESTERASE REACTION

With Fluoride Inhibition

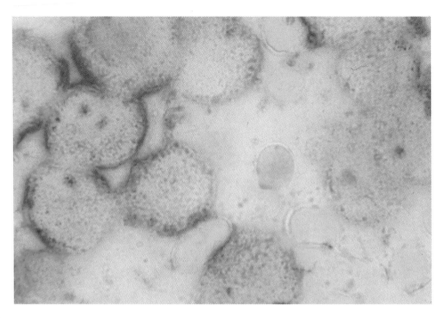

Figure IC1-4   Negative for inhibition.

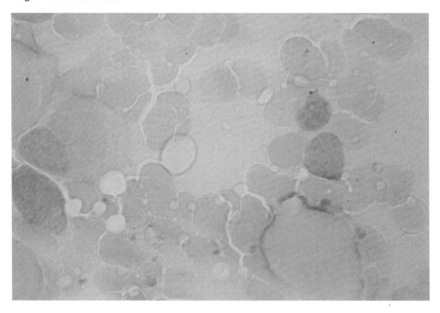

Figure IC1-5   Positive for inhibition.

Cell Type

Monocytic line

Description

Megakaryocytes, histiocytes, and macrophages demonstrate positivity
Lymphocytes may have a punctate red product
Monocytes are sensitive to fluoride inhibition and will not show positivity
1+ positivity in granulocytic series

Clinical Conditions

■ Acute myelomonocytic (M4) and monocytic (M5) leukemias are inhibited by fluoride
■ Acute lymphocytic leukemia or leukemias of granulocytic origins are not inhibited

Without Fluoride Inhibition

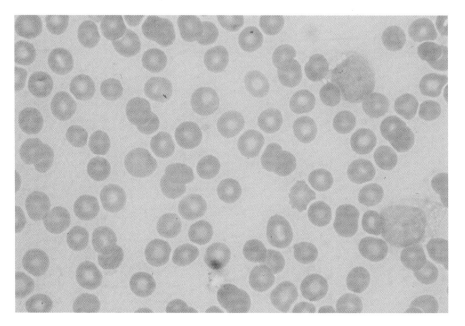

Figure **IC1-6**   Negative

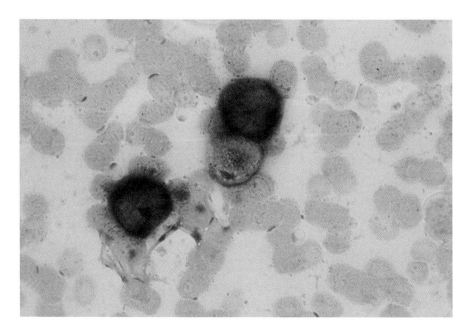

Figure **IC1-7**   Positive

Cell Type

Monocytic line

Description

Megakaryocytes, histiocytes, and macrophages demonstrate positivity
Lymphocytes may have a punctate positivity
Monocytes are sensitive to fluoride inhibition and will not show positivity

Clinical Conditions

■ Acute myelomonocytic (M4) and monocytic (M5) leukemias are inhibited by fluoride
■ Acute lymphocytic leukemia or leukemias of granulocytic origins are not inhibited

Specific Esterase Reaction

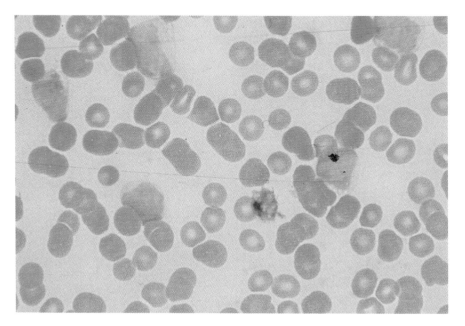

Figure **IC1-8**   Negative

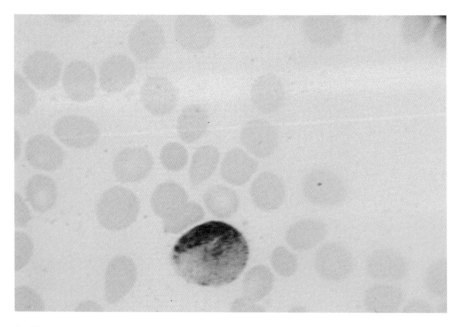

Figure **IC1-9**   Positive

Cell Type

Some myeloblasts, promyelocytes, myelocytes, metamyelocytes, bands, segmented
neutrophils, and abnormal eosinophils

Description

Esterases are enzymes that are capable of hydrolyzing the aliphatic and aromatic
ester bonds of the substrate naphthol AS-D chloroacetate
Produces a positive reaction, indicated by red to magenta color

Clinical Conditions

■ Differentiates granulocytes from lymphocytes and monocytes
■ Acute myelocytic leukemia without maturation (M1)
■ Acute myelocytic leukemia with maturation (M2)
■ Acute promyelocytic leukemia (M3)
■ Acute myelomonocytic leukemia (M4)
■ Acute myelomonocytic leukemia with abnormal bone marrow eosinophils

Combined Esterase Reaction

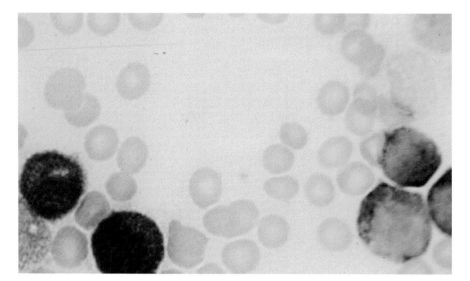

Figure **IC1-10**

Positive

Cell Type

Differentiation of granulocytic and monocytic series

Description

Both alpha-naphthyl acetate (nonspecific) and naphthyl chloroacetate(specific) are
used as substrates

Monocytic series demonstrates positivity with the nonspecific esterase

Granulocytic series demonstrates a positive reaction with the specific esterase (color
depends on couplers used)

Clinical Conditions

- Acute myelomonocytic leukemia (M4)—demonstrates the coexpression of
  neutrophilic and monocytic enzymes
- Acute monoblastic leukemia (M5a)
- Acute monocytic leukemia (M5b)

Iron Stain—Prussian Blue Reaction

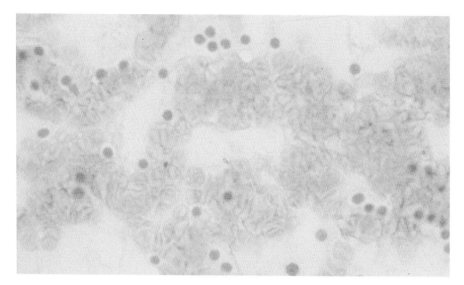

Figure **IC1-11**   Negative

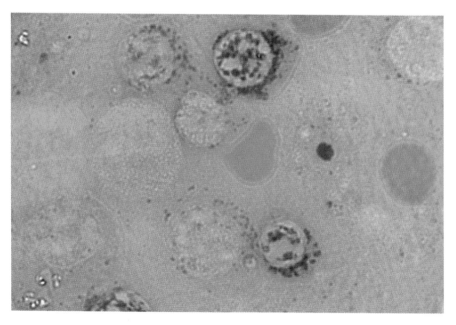

Figure **IC1-12**   Positive

Cell Type

Erythroblasts, erythrocytes, macrophages, histiocytes

Description

Iron in the form of hemosiderin is normally present in developing normoblasts and in the reticuloendothelial cells of the bone marrow. A Prussian blue color is produced when ferric iron of hemosiderin reacts with an acid ferrocyanide solution to form ferric ferrocyanide.

Positivity or the presence of iron is indicated by the presence of blue to blue-green granules

May be used to determine the presence of iron stores in the marrow

May be used to demonstrate increased numbers of sideroblasts or the presence of pathologic ferric iron located in mitochondria of the erythroblast (ringed sideroblast)

Clinical Conditions

- Myelodysplastic syndromes
- Acute erythroleukemia (M6)
- Thalassemias
- Intramacrophage iron is decreased in iron deficiency and increased in hemochromatosis and chronic diseases

ACID ELUTION (KLEIHAUER-BETKE STAIN)

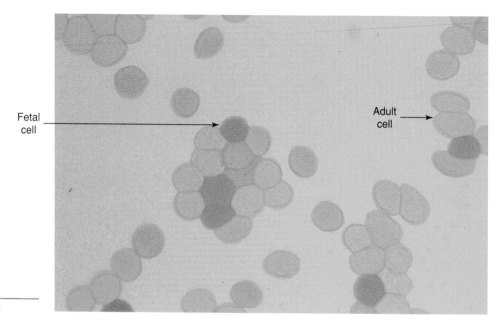

Fetal cell

Adult cell

Figure IC1-13

Cell Type

Red blood cells

Description

Cells containing hemoglobin F will appear pink to red
Cells containing no hemoglobin F will have only their outer membrane visible
    (ghost cells)

Clinical Conditions

■ Hereditary persistence of fetal hemoglobin
■ Myelodysplastic syndromes
■ Some leukemias

Leukocyte Alkaline Phosphatase Stain

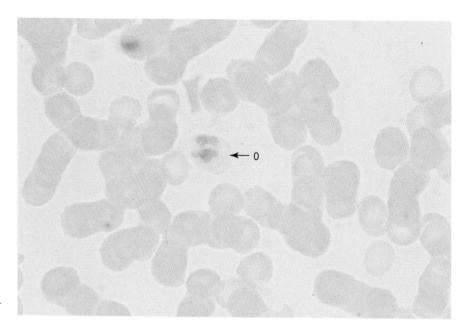

Figure **IC1-14**

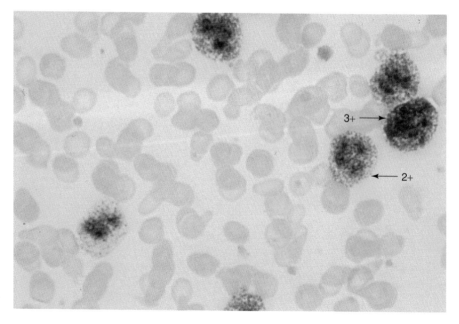

Figure **IC1-15**

Cell Type

Granulocyte distinguishes leukemoid reaction from chronic myelogenous leukemia

Description

LAP is an enzyme associated with the specific granules
Presence of leukocyte alkaline phosphatase activity indicates intracellular metabolic activity
Positivity is indicated by either a ruby red color or a blue-purple color
Positivity is quantitated
100 consecutive bands or segmented neutrophils are scored using the following criteria:
  0 Colorless
  1 Diffuse positivity; occasional granules
  2 Diffuse positivity; moderate numbers of granules
  3 Strong positivity; numerous granules
  4 Very strong positivity; dark, confluent granules
The scores of the 100 cells are summed

Clinical Conditions

Increased:

■ Leukemoid reaction
■ Polycythemia vera
■ Pregnancy
■ Infections
■ Chronic myelocytic leukemia blast crisis
■ Myelofibrosis

Decreased:

■ Chronic myelogenous leukemia
■ Paroxysmal nocturnal hemoglobinuria
■ Some myelodysplastic syndromes

New Methylene Blue and Brilliant Cresyl Blue Stains

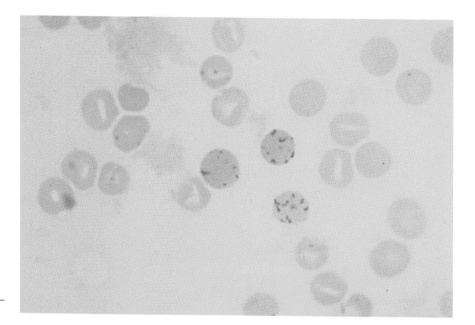

Figure **IC1-16**

Cell Type

Red blood cells

Description

Supravital stains commonly used in demonstrating aggregates of RNA in immature
   erythrocytes (reticulocytes)
Pappenheimer bodies, Howell-Jolly bodies, and Heinz bodies are also stained

Clinical Conditions

- Hemolytic anemias
- Folate deficiency
- Vitamin B_{12} deficiency
- Glucose-6-phosphate dehydrogenase deficiency
- Hb H disease
- Myelodysplastic syndromes

Periodic Acid-Schiff Reaction

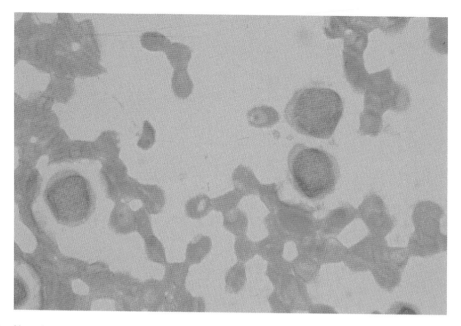

Figure **IC1-17**   Negative

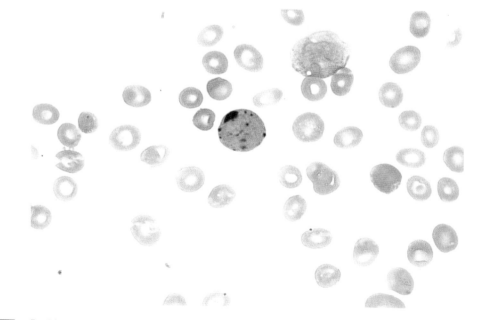

Figure **IC1-18**   Positive

Cell Type

Neoplastic erythroblasts, granulocytes, monocytes, lymphoblasts, and
    megakaryocytes (most hematopoietic cells in variable quantities)

Description

PAS stains glycogen
Positivity is indicated by a bright pink color
Lymphocytes, granulocytes, monocytes, and megakaryocytes may be positive
Normal erythroblasts are negative

Clinical Conditions

- Acute erythroleukemia (positive)
- Thalassemia, iron deficiency, sideroblastic anemia (may be positive)
- Burkitt lymphoma cells (negative) (L3)
- Acute lymphocytic leukemia (may have block positivity) (L1, L2)
- Any severe dyserythropoiesis
- Acute myelomonocytic leukemia with abnormal bone marrow eosinophils
  (granules are positive)

Peroxidase Stain

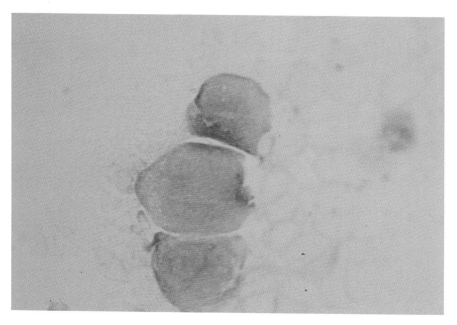

Figure IC1-19   Negative

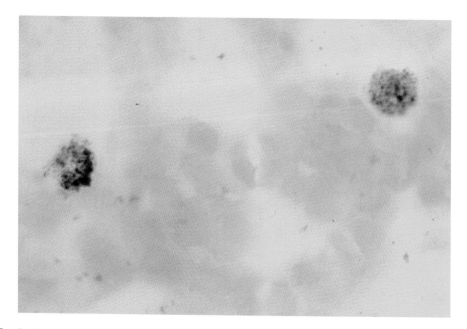

Figure IC1-20   Positive

Cell Type

Myeloid cells—primary granules of the neutrophilic and eosinophilic series, monocytes are faintly positive

Description

Myeloperoxidase is an enzyme capable of oxidizing dye substrates in the presence of hydrogen peroxide

Positivity is indicated by the presence of black or red-brown granules (color depends on the substrate)

Positivity is found in some myeloblasts, promyelocytes, myelocytes, metamyelocytes, neutrophils, eosinophils, and faintly positive in monocytes

Early myeloblasts, basophils, plasma cells, and lymphocytic cells and erythroid cells are negative

Clinical Conditions

■ Acute myelocytic leukemia without maturation (M1)
■ Acute myelocytic leukemia with maturation (M2)
■ Acute promyelocytic leukemia (M3)
■ Acute myelomonocytic leukemia (M4)
■ Erythroleukemia (M6a)

Sudan Black B Stain

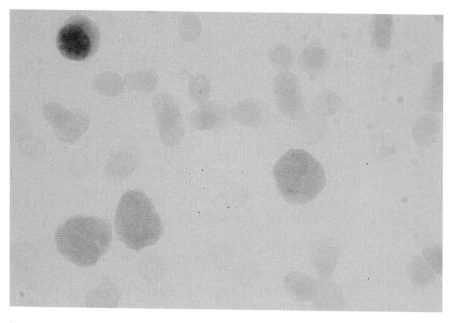

Figure IC1-21   Negative

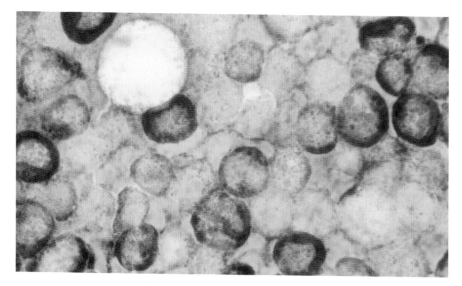

Figure IC1-22   Positive

Cell Type

Neutrophilic and eosinophilic cells and their precursors, monocytes are weakly positive

Description

Separates AML from acute lymphocytic leukemia (ALL)

Sudan black B stains lipid particles found in primary and secondary granules, as well as giving a weak positivity in lysosomal granules found in the monocytic cells

Lymphocytes may rarely have these granules

Positivity is indicated by a brownish-black–colored granule

Clinical Conditions

- Acute myelocytic leukemia without maturation (M1)
- Acute myelocytic leukemia with maturation (M2)
- Acute promyelocytic leukemia (M3)
- Acute myelomonocytic leukemia (M4)
- Acute monoblastic leukemia (M5a) (if myeloblasts are present)
- Acute monocytic leukemia (M5b) (if myeloblasts are present)
- Erythroleukemia (M6a) (if myeloblasts are present)

Terminal Deoxynucleotidyl Transferase Reaction

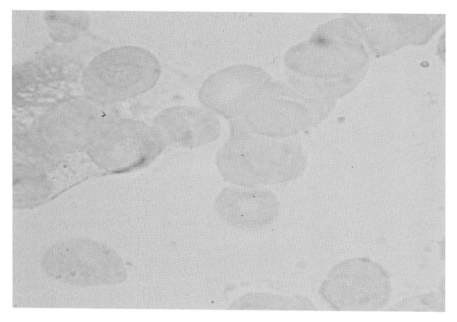

Figure **IC1-23**   Negative

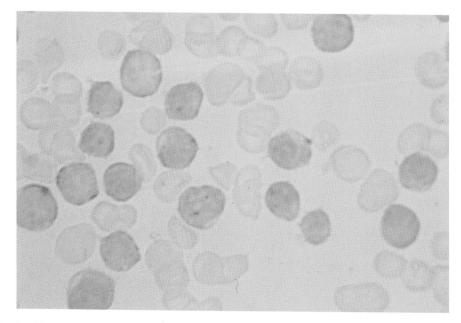

Figure **IC1-24**   Positive

Cell Type

Primitive lymphocytic cells and neoplastic cells

Description

Enzyme (DNA polymerase) found in the nucleus
Demonstrated through immunofluorescent or immunoperoxidase procedures
Positivity is demonstrated by a lime-green fluorescence or red to brownish-red
  staining

Clinical Conditions

- T-cell acute lymphoblastic leukemia
- Precursor B-cell acute lymphocytic leukemia
- Undifferentiated leukemia (small % positive)
- Chronic myelocytic leukemia with blast crisis (small % positive)
- Lymphoblastic lymphoma
- Chronic myelocytic leukemia with lymphoblastic transformation

Toluidine Blue Stain

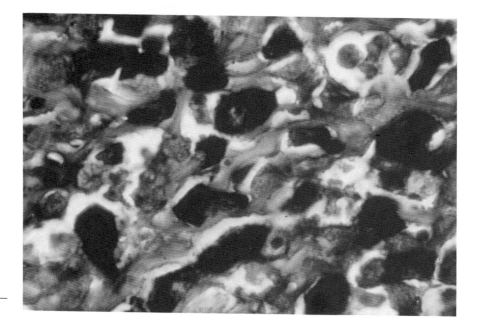

Figure IC1-25

Cell Type

Basophils and mast cells

Description

Reacts with acid mucopolysaccharides (heparan sulfate) to form metachromatic
  granules
Positivity is indicated by a red-violet color
May not be positive in neoplastic disorders involving these cells

Clinical Conditions

■ Mast cell disease
■ Basophilic leukemias

Unit II

Hematologic Disorders

- **Section A.** Red Blood Cell Disorders

- **Section B.** White Blood Cell Disorders

- **Section C.** Miscellaneous Disorders

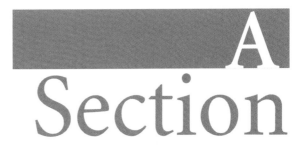

A

Section

Red Blood Cell Disorders

CHAPTER

1

Erythrocytosis

POLYCYTHEMIA VERA

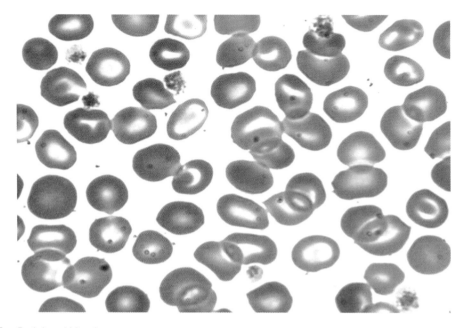

Figure **IIA1-1**   Peripheral blood smear.

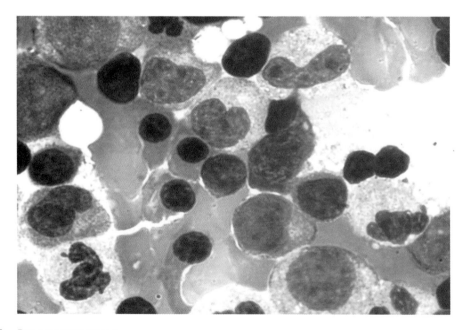

Figure **IIA1-2**   Bone marrow smear.

Clinical Features

- Usually diagnosed in persons aged 55–70 years
- Slight male predominance
- Headache, confusion, altered mental status, dizziness, visual changes, tinnitus, paresthesias
- Weight loss, epigastric pain, gout, pruritus, thrombosis, and hemorrhage
- Plethora, hypertension, and a mild to moderate degree of splenomegaly and hepatomegaly

Pathology

- Malignancy
- Excessive bone marrow production of red blood cells and an increase in total red blood cell volume
- White blood cell and platelet counts may also increase to a lesser extent
- Increased blood viscosity
- Thrombosis is a complication in more than half of the cases
- Myelofibrosis or acute myeloid leukemia may develop
- Polycythemic stage
- Increased red blood cell mass
- "Spent" phase and postpolycythemic myelofibrosis and myeloid metaplasia
- Anemia
- Bone marrow fibrosis
- Extramedullary hematopoiesis
- Hypersplenism

Laboratory Features

White Blood Cells

- Increased in about two-thirds of patients
- Immature forms usually not seen
- Eosinophils and basophils may be increased
- Leukocyte alkaline phosphatase increased in three-quarters of cases

Platelets

- Normal to increased

Red Blood Cells

- Hemoglobin level increased
- Hematocrit level increased
- Red blood cell mass increased

Bone Marrow

- Hyperplastic
- Erythroid hyperplasia
- Increased megakaryocytes
- Granulocytic hyperplasia
- Increased reticulin in postpolycythemic myelofibrosis and myeloid metaplasia
- Iron stores are often depleted

Traditional Criteria for Diagnosis

Meet three major criteria or two major and two minor criteria
Major criteria

- Increased red blood cell mass
- Splenomegaly
- Normal oxygen level

Minor criteria

- Platelet count $>400 \times 10^9$/L
- White blood cell count $>12 \times 10^9$/L
- Elevated leukocyte alkaline phosphate level
- Elevated vitamin B_{12} level or unbound vitamin B_{12} binding capacity

Another Traditional Criteria for Diagnosis

Meet three major criteria or two major and two minor criteria
Major criteria

- Elevated red blood cell mass
- Normal oxygen level
- Splenomegaly

Minor criteria

- Thrombocytosis
- Neutrophil leukocytosis
- Positive endogenous erythroid colony assay or low serum erythropoietin level

World Health Organization Criteria for Diagnosis

Elevated red blood cell mass
No identified cause of secondary erythrocytosis
Plus one of the following:

■ Splenomegaly
■ Clonal abnormality, excluding Ph chromosome or BCR/ALB fusion gene
■ In vivo formation of endogenous erythroid colony

Or any two of the following:

■ Platelet count $>400 \times 10^9$/L
■ White blood cell count $>12 \times 10^9$/L
■ Panmyelosis of the bone marrow with prominent erythroid and megakaryocytic proliferation
■ Low serum erythropoietin levels

Diagnostic Scheme

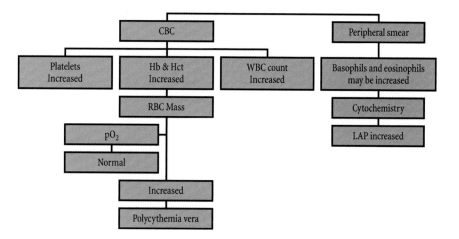

RELATIVE POLYCYTHEMIA (GAISBOCK SYNDROME)

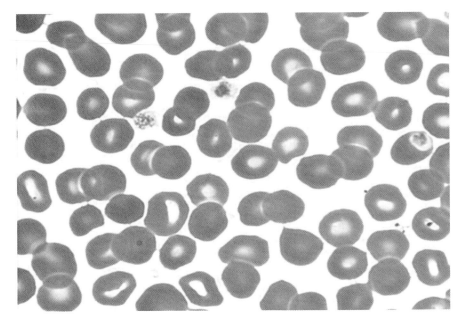

Peripheral blood smear.

Clinical Features

- Usually occurs in males aged 45–55 years
- The patients tend to be obese, have hypertension, and are heavy smokers

Pathology

- Normal red blood cell mass and clearly decreased plasma volume
- Red blood cell mass at the upper range of normal; plasma volume at the lower range of normal
- Cause of the low plasma volume is not understood but may be related to a variety of causes, including emotional stress, alcoholism, heavy smoking, chronic anxiety, and hypertension

Laboratory Features

White Blood Cells

■ Not remarkable

Platelets

■ Not remarkable

Red Blood Cells

■ Hemoglobin level increased
■ Hematocrit level increased
■ Red blood cell count increased
■ Red blood cell mass normal
■ Plasma volume decreased
■ Oxygen pressure normal
■ Erythropoietin level normal

Diagnostic Scheme

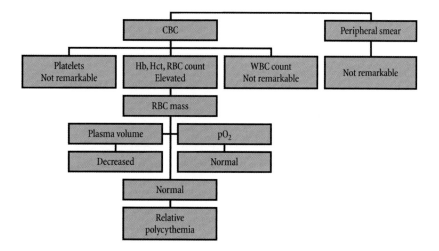

SECONDARY POLYCYTHEMIA

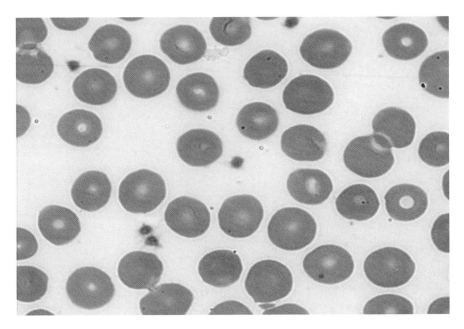

Figure IIA1-4   Peripheral blood smear.

Clinical Features

■ Related to the actual cause of the erythrocytosis
■ May include plethora, headache, dizziness, visual disturbances, fatigue, paresthesias, decreased mental acuity, obesity, and daytime sleepiness

Pathology

- May be secondary to conditions where there is decreased delivery of oxygen to the tissues, which results in the release of erythropoietin—appropriate secretion of erythropoietin
- May occur in conditions in which delivery of oxygen to the tissues is normal—inappropriate secretion of erythropoietin
- Conditions associated with appropriate secretion of erythropoietin
  - Living at a high altitude
  - High-affinity hemoglobins (e.g., Hb Chesapeake, Rainier, Capetown, Bethesda)
  - Carbon monoxide poisoning
  - Obstructive sleep apnea
  - Drug induced (e.g., testosterone)
  - Obesity-hypoventilation syndrome (Pickwickian)
- Conditions associated with inappropriate secretion of erythropoietin
  - Hepatoma
  - Pheochromocytoma
  - Renal cell cancer, renal cyst, or renal artery stenosis
  - Cerebellar hemangioma

Laboratory Features

White Blood Cells

- Not remarkable

Platelets

- Not remarkable

Red Blood Cells

- Hemoglobin level increased
- Hematocrit level increased
- Red blood cell count increased
- Red blood cell mass increased
- Increased erythropoietin
- Decreased oxygen pressure if due to anoxia; normal oxygen pressure if due to tumor

Diagnostic Scheme

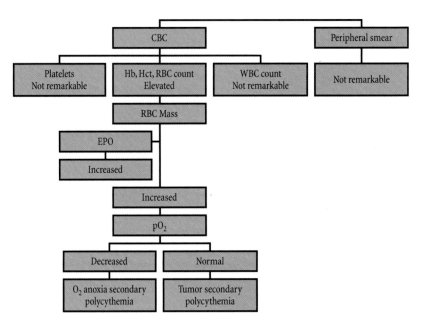

CHAPTER

2

Hypochromic Anemias

αTHALASSEMIA (4 GENE DELETION)

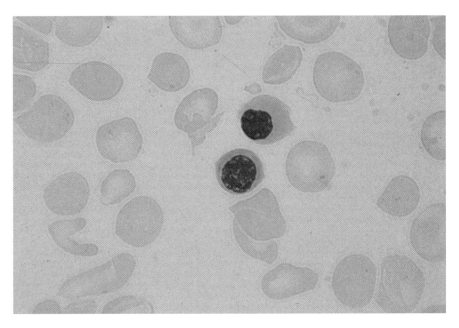

Figure IIA2-1   Cord blood smear.

Clinical Features

■ Produces hydrops fetalis, and affected infants are either stillborn or die within hours of birth
■ Marked hepatosplenomegaly
■ Marked anemia

Pathology

■ Parents are usually heterozygous for α thalassemia ($-/\alpha\alpha$)
■ No α chains are produced ($-/-$)
■ Free γ chains form tetrads, producing hemoglobin
■ Bart's hemoglobin
■ Excess β chains form tetramers and inclusions in red blood cells, which shortens survival

Laboratory Features

White Blood Cells

- Not remarkable

Platelets

- Not remarkable

Red Blood Cells

- Macrocytic/hypochromic anemia
- Mean corpuscular hemoglobin level decreased
- Mean corpuscular volume increased
- Increased nucleated red blood cells
- 80–90% Bart's hemoglobin
- 10–20% Portland hemoglobin
- Trace of hemoglobin H

Diagnostic Scheme

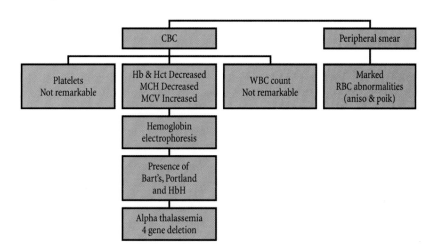

α THALASSEMIA (3 GENE DELETION—HEMOGLOBIN H DISEASE)

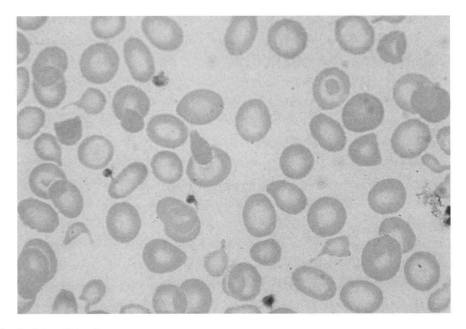

Figure **IIA2-2**   Peripheral blood smear.

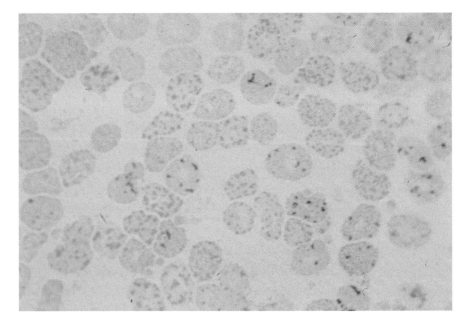

Figure **IIA2-3**   Brilliant cresyl blue stain.

Clinical Features

- Splenomegaly
- Variable anemia, more severe during pregnancy, infections, and exposure to oxidant drugs

Pathology

- Deletion of three α genes $(-/-\alpha)$
  - Reduced hemoglobin A and thus oxygen delivery
- Excess unpaired β chains are present and form unstable tetramers (β_4) (hemoglobin H)
  - Hemoglobin H has high oxygen affinity, resulting in decreased oxygen delivery
- Tetramers can cause disturbances in red blood cell metabolism, membrane function, and deformability, resulting in chronic hemolytic anemia

Laboratory Features

White Blood Cells

- Not remarkable

Platelets

- Not remarkable

Red Blood Cells

- Hemoglobin level, 8.0–10.0 g/dL
- Reticulocyte count, 5–10% of red blood cells
- Microcytic/hypochromic anemia
- Increased red blood cell distribution width
- Poikilocytosis
- Polychromasia

Diagnostic Scheme

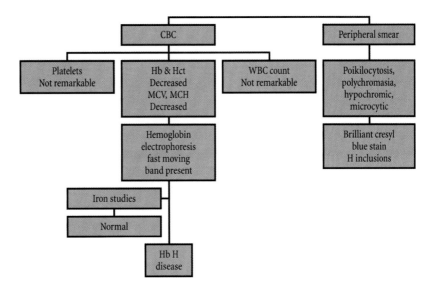

α THALASSEMIA MINOR AND SILENT CARRIER

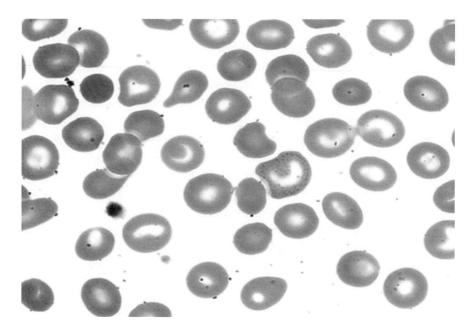

Figure IIA2-4   Peripheral blood smear.

Clinical Features

■ No clinical disease is seen with either the trait or the silent carrier

Pathology

Minor or Trait

■ Decreased production of α-globin chains
■ Exists in two forms:
   ■ Heterozygous α^0 thalassemia ($-/\alpha\alpha$)
   ■ Homozygous α^+ thalassemia ($-\alpha/-\alpha$)
■ Both forms are common in Southeast Asians, Chinese, and Filipinos
■ Homozygous form is common in African Americans (about 3%)

Silent Carrier

■ Heterozygous α^+ ($-\alpha/\alpha\alpha$) is common in Southeast Asians, Chinese, and Filipinos
■ About 28% of African Americans have the heterozygous α^+ thalassemia

Laboratory Features

Minor or Trait

White Blood Cells

- Not remarkable

Platelets

- Not remarkable

Red Blood Cells

- Microcytic and slightly hypochromic anemia
- Poikilocytosis
- Codocytes
- Normal or slightly increased red blood cell distribution width
- Hemoglobin H inclusions may occasionally be found in brilliant cresyl blue (BCB) prep
- 5–15% Bart's hemoglobin in cord blood (normal after about age 3 months)

Silent Carrier

White Blood Cells

- Not remarkable

Platelets

- Not remarkable

Red Blood Cells

- No hematologic manifestations
- 1–2% Bart's hemoglobin found at birth
- Rare hemoglobin H inclusion found in BCB prep

Diagnostic Scheme

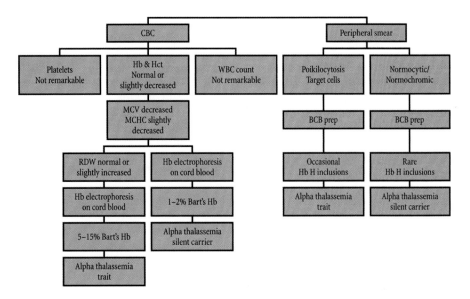

ANEMIA OF CHRONIC DISEASE

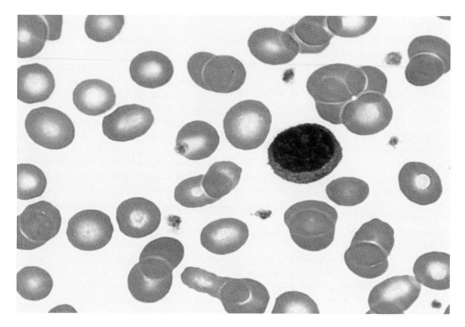

Peripheral blood smear.

Clinical Features

■ Those of the underlying disease: inflammatory, neoplastic, or infectious state

Pathology

■ Hypoproliferative anemia
■ Impaired release of iron from the reticuloendothelial cells for hemoglobin synthesis
■ Decreased red blood cell survival

Laboratory Features

White Blood Cells

■ Not consistent—depends on the underlying disease

Platelets

■ Not consistent—depends on the underlying disease

Red Blood Cells

■ Decreased hemoglobin and hematocrit
■ Normocytic/normochromic anemia
■ Microcytic/hypochromic anemia
■ Reticulocyte count normal to slightly increased

Bone Marrow

■ Normal to increased hemosiderin
■ Decreased sideroblasts
■ Decreased serum iron level
■ Normal or decreased total iron binding capacity
■ Decreased % saturation (usually >15%)
■ Normal or increased serum ferritin level

Diagnostic Scheme

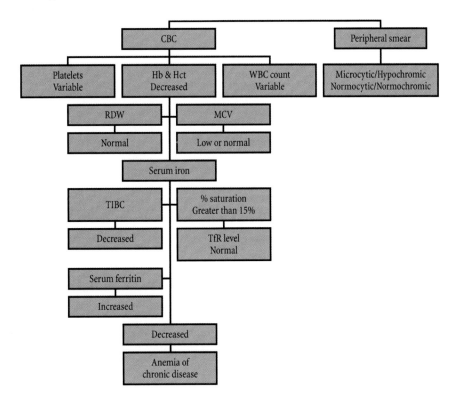

β THALASSEMIA

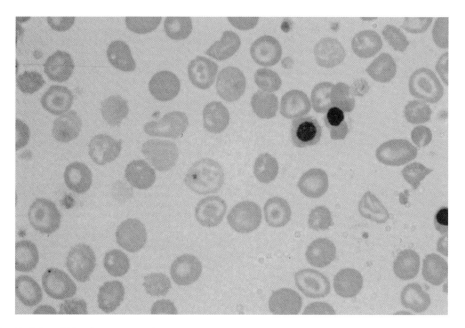

Figure IIA2-6   Peripheral blood smear—major.

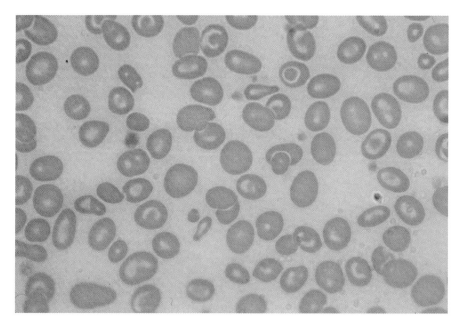

Figure IIA2-7   Peripheral blood smear—intermedia.

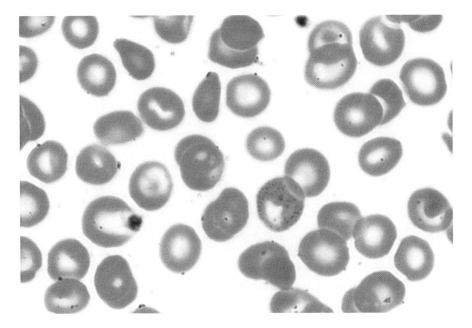

Figure **IIA2-8**   Peripheral blood smear—minor.

Clinical Features

- Major variant
    - Severe anemia
    - Transfusion dependent
    - Growth retardation
    - Massive hepatosplenomegaly
    - Severe ineffective erythropoiesis
    - Early death with iron overload
- Intermedia variant
    - Moderate anemia
    - Splenomegaly
    - Moderate, ineffective erythropoiesis
- Minor variant
    - Mild anemia
    - Usually no symptoms

Pathology

- β chain production is absent or diminished—the more β chain produced, the less severe the disease
- Unmatched α chains accumulate and aggregate
  - Ineffective erythropoiesis
  - Chronic hemolytic process
- Decreased erythrocyte hemoglobin production

Laboratory Features

White Blood Cells

- Not remarkable

Platelets

- Not remarkable

Red Blood Cells

- Nucleated red blood cells on peripheral smear (found in major and intermedia)
- Hypochromic/microcytic anemia
- Target cells present
- Distorted cells
- Basophilic stippling
- Normal to increased red blood cell distribution width
- Increased red blood cell count relative to hemoglobin and hematocrit

Bone Marrow

- Ineffective erythropoiesis because of the accumulation of α-globulin chains
- Extremely hyperplastic

Hemoglobin Electrophoresis

- Only hemoglobin F and hemoglobin A_2 are found in β^0 thalassemia
- Small amounts of hemoglobin A may be found in β^+ thalassemia
- Increased hemoglobin A_2 is indicative of β thalassemia

Diagnostic Scheme

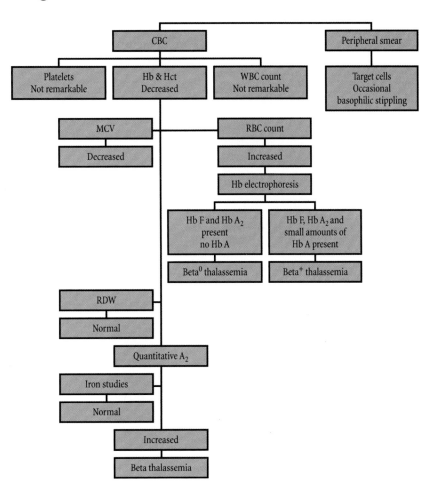

ERYTHROPOIETIC PORPHYRIA (GUNTHER'S DISEASE)

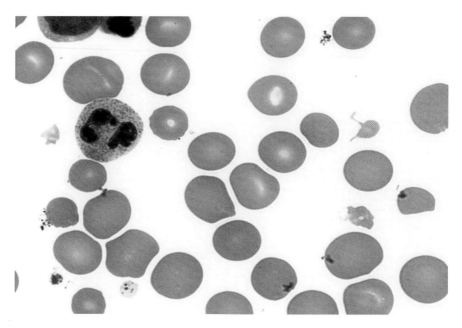

Figure IIA2-9   Peripheral blood smear.

Clinical Features

- Rare autosomal recessive disease
- Appears in infancy
- Urine is pink to reddish-brown
- Vesicular or bullous eruptions appear on exposed areas of the body
- Scarring occurs and may lead to severe deformities of the nose, ears, eyes, and fingers
- Teeth fluoresce
- Hypertrichosis affects the entire body
- Splenomegaly

Pathology

- Decreased tissue uroporphyrinogen III cosynthetase
- Hemolytic anemia

Laboratory Features

White Blood Cells

■ Not remarkable

Platelets

■ Not remarkable

Red Blood Cells

■ Moderate to severe normocytic/normochromic anemia
■ Polychromatophilia
■ Nucleated red blood cells in the peripheral blood
■ Red blood cells fluoresce
■ Increased reticulocyte count
■ Excessive porphyrin deposits in the red blood cells

Bone Marrow

■ Erythroid hyperplasia
■ Normoblasts fluoresce
■ Ineffective erythropoiesis

Chemistries

■ Normal serum iron level
■ Normal serum ferritin level
■ Increased unconjugated bilirubin level
■ Increased urine and fecal urobilinogen levels
■ Excessive amounts of uroporphyrin I and coproporphyrin I in urine and feces

Diagnostic Scheme

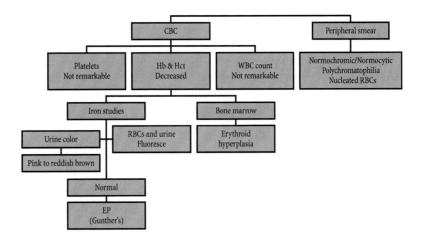

ERYTHROPOIETIC PROTOPORPHYRIA

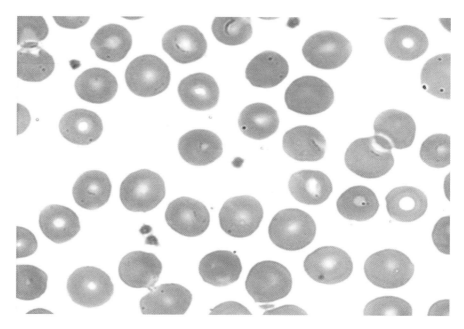

Figure IIA2-10   Peripheral blood smear.

Clinical Features

- Autosomal dominant or recessive transmission
- Usually begins before teen years
- Burning, redness, itching, swelling of skin
- Photosensitivity is not severe
- Relatively mild course

Pathology

- Deficiency of ferrochelatase
- Accumulation of protoporphyrin

Laboratory Features

White Blood Cells

- Not remarkable

Platelets

- Not remarkable

Red Blood Cells

- No hemolytic anemia
- No abnormalities
- Red blood cells may accumulate protoporphyrins and fluoresce

Bone Marrow

- No abnormalities
- The cytoplasm of normoblasts fluoresce intensely

Chemistries

- Increased levels of protoporphyrin found in red blood cells, plasma, and feces but not in urine

Diagnostic Scheme

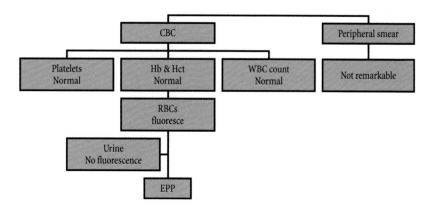

HEMOGLOBIN CONSTANT SPRING SYNDROME

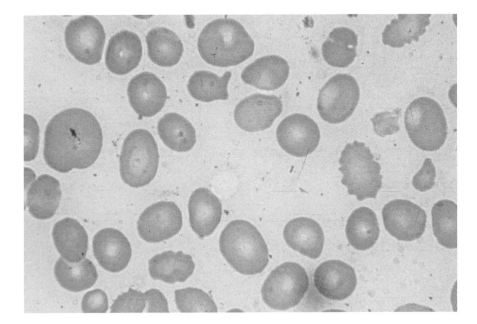

Figure IIA2-11   Peripheral blood smear.

Clinical Features

- Homozygotes have a condition similar to mild α thalassemia—mild anemia, mild jaundice, splenomegaly
- Heterozygotes usually have no clinical abnormalities
- Common in Thailand, Chinese, and Greek ancestry with α thalassemia syndromes
- May occur in about 40% of hemoglobin H disease in Southeast Asians

Pathology

- Four different types of hemoglobins
- Hemoglobin Constant Spring is formed from the combination of two structurally abnormal α chains, each elongated by 31 amino acids at the C-terminal end and two normal β chains
- The abnormal α chains are inefficiently synthesized owing to reduced stability of the messenger RNA translation apparatus
- The deficiency of α chain synthesis produces an α thalassemia–like syndrome

Laboratory Features

White Blood Cells

■ Not remarkable

Platelets

■ Not remarkable

Red Blood Cells

■ Mild microcytic, hypochromic anemia
■ Hemoglobin level usually 9.0–11.0 g/dL
■ Reticulocyte count, 3.5–7.5%
■ Anisocytosis, poikilocytosis
■ Codocytes

Hemoglobin Electrophoresis (Cellulose Acetate, pH 8.4)

■ Migrates on the cathode side of hemoglobin A_2
■ In homozygotes
  ■ Bart's hemoglobin present at birth
  ■ Hemoglobin Constant Spring 5–7%
  ■ Hemoglobins A_2 and F normal
■ In heterozygotes
  ■ Hemoglobin Constant Spring 0.2–1.7%

Diagnostic Scheme

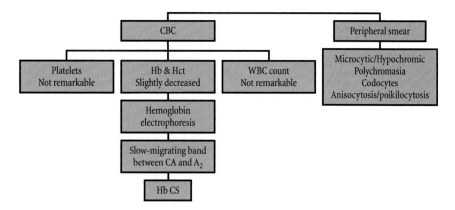

HEMOGLOBIN LEPORE SYNDROME

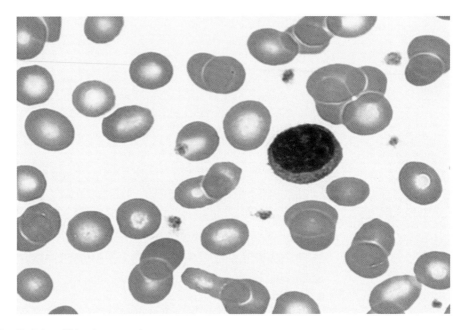

Figure **IIA2-12**   Peripheral blood smear—heterozygous.

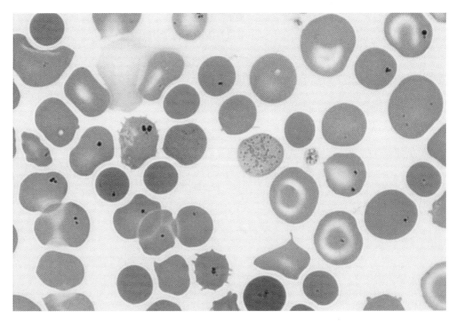

Figure **IIA2-13**   Peripheral blood smear—homozygous.

Clinical Features

- Common in middle and eastern Europe
- Homozygotes
  - Described as a condition that resembles thalassemia intermedia
  - Variable anemia depending on racial group
  - Symptoms develop with the first 5 years of life
  - Hepatosplenomegaly is significant
  - Skeletal abnormalities may exist also with growth retardation
- Heterozygotes
  - Mild anemia and the condition resembles thalassemia minor
  - May be asymptomatic
  - Slight splenomegaly

Pathology

- The non–α hemoglobin chain is a λ-β–globin hybrid in which the N-terminal end of the λ chain is fused to the C-terminal end of a β chain
- Believed to arise during meiosis from aberrant recombination of misaligned λ and β chains on separate chromosomes
- Two hybrid chains combine with two α chains to form hemoglobin Lepore
- Hemoglobin Lepore is stable and has normal functional properties, except a slight increase in oxygen
- The abnormal chains are ineffectively synthesized, leading to an excess of α chains that precipitate, leading to cell membrane damage in inflexibility—hemolytic anemia is the result

Laboratory Features

Homozygotes

- Hemoglobin level is usually 4.0–11.0 g/dL
- Microcytic, hypochromic anemia
- Anisocytosis poikilocytosis, codocytes, basophilic stippling, Pappenheimer bodies

Heterozygotes

- Hemoglobin level is slightly decreased
- Microcytic, hypochromic anemia

Bone Marrow

- Erythroid marrow expands and produces abnormal cells
- Ineffective erythropoiesis contributes to the anemia as the abnormal cells are destroyed

Hemoglobin Electrophoresis (Cellulose Acetate, pH 8.4)

- Homozygotes
  - 0% hemoglobin A
  - 0% hemoglobin A_2
  - 75% hemoglobin F
  - 25% hemoglobin Lepore (hemoglobin Lepore migrates like hemoglobin S)
- Heterozygotes
  - 75–85% hemoglobin A
  - About 2% hemoglobin A_2
  - 1–6% hemoglobin F
  - 7–15% hemoglobin Lepore

Diagnostic Scheme

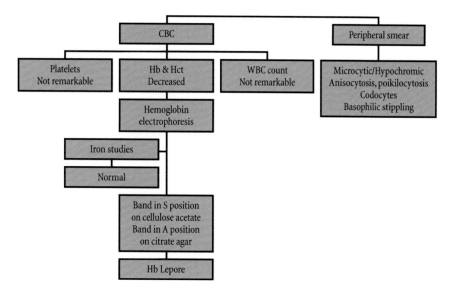

HEREDITARY PERSISTENCE OF FETAL HEMOGLOBIN

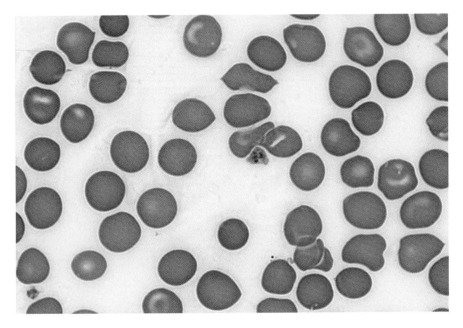

Figure IIA2-14   Peripheral blood smear.

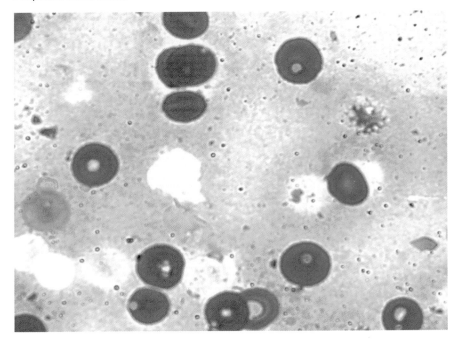

Figure IIA2-15   Kleihauer-Betke stain.

Clinical Features

■ Usually no or minimal anemia
■ In the homozygous state, there are no findings suggestive of thalassemia (abnormal growth, splenomegaly)

Pathology

■ Deletion/inactivation of λ and β genes
■ Absence of λ and β chain synthesis is compensated for by increased γ chain production into adult life, causing the increased levels of hemoglobin F
■ Two types exist:
  ■ Pancellular (Black, Greek)
  ■ Heterocellular (Swiss)
■ Hemoglobin F has normal to slightly higher oxygen affinity; thus, patients are usually asymptomatic
■ Slightly increased oxygen affinity will lead to increased erythropoiesis

Laboratory Features

White Blood Cells

■ Not remarkable

Platelets

■ Not remarkable

Red Blood Cells

■ Microcytic/hypochromic anemia
■ Mild erythrocytosis
■ Mean corpuscular volume decreased
■ Anisocytosis
■ Poikilocytosis
■ Target cells present

Hemoglobin Electrophoresis

■ Homozygotes
  ■ 100% hemoglobin F
■ Heterozygotes
  ■ 10–30% hemoglobin F
  ■ 1–2% hemoglobin A_2

Diagnostic Scheme

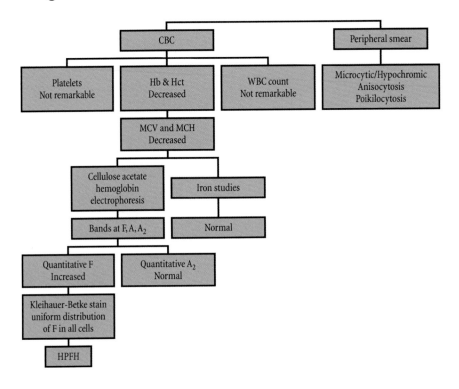

IRON DEFICIENCY ANEMIA

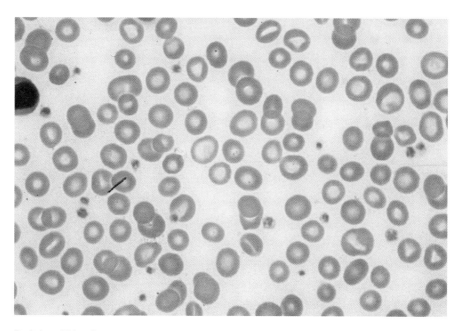

Figure IIA2-16   Peripheral blood smear.

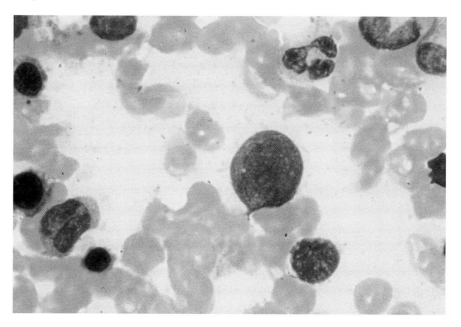

Figure IIA2-17   Bone marrow smear.

Clinical Features

- Fatigue, loss of stamina, exercise intolerance
- Delayed growth
- Lethargy
- Dizziness
- Pallor
- Glossitis
- Koilonychia (spoon-nails)
- Crave dirt or paint (pica) or ice (pagophagia)

Pathology

- Deficient heme synthesis
- Ineffective erythropoiesis
- Increased iron loss
  - Pregnancy
  - Menstruation
  - Chronic blood loss from gastrointestinal tract
- Low availability of iron
  - Rapid growth period
  - Defective gastric function
  - Achlorhydria
  - Gastrectomy

Laboratory Features

White Blood Cells

- Not remarkable

Platelets

- Normal or slightly increased

Red Blood Cells

- Hemoglobin and hematocrit levels decreased
- Microcytic/hypochromic anemia
- Reticulocyte count normal or slightly increased
- Increased red blood cell distribution width
- Pencil- or cigar-shaped red blood cells, codocytes

Bone Marrow

■ Normoblastic hyperplasia
■ Absent hemosiderin
■ Decreased sideroblasts (<10%)
■ Normoblasts are smaller than normal, with ragged rims of cytoplasm containing little hemoglobin

Chemistries

■ Decreased serum iron level
■ Increased total iron binding capacity
■ Decreased % saturation (<15%)
■ Decreased serum ferritin level
■ Increased zinc protoporphyrin

Diagnostic Scheme

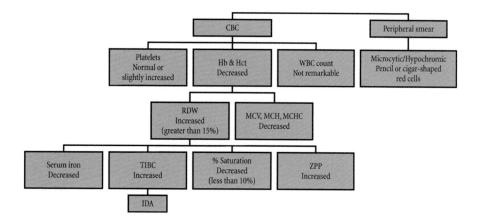

LEAD INTOXICATION (PLUMBISM)

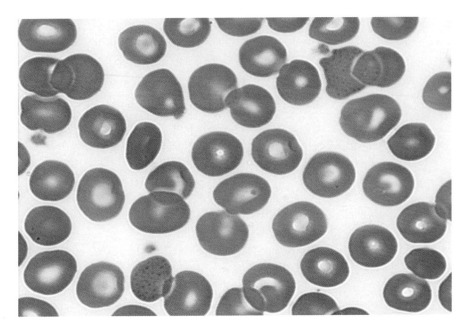

Figure **IIA2-18**   Peripheral blood smear.

Clinical Features

- Abdominal pain
- Constipation
- Vomiting
- Muscle weakness
- Lead line on gums
- Skin lesions
- Neurologic dysfunctions

Pathology

- Synthesis of α- and β-globin chains is impaired
- Interference with iron storage in the mitochondria, which may lead to sideroblastic anemia
- Activity of most enzymes in heme synthesis is inhibited
- Ineffective erythropoiesis (hemolysis because of RNA breakdown)

Laboratory Features

White Blood Cells

■ Not consistent findings

Platelets

■ Not remarkable

Red Blood Cells

■ Microcytic/hypochromic anemia
■ Basophilic stippling
■ Reticulocyte count normal to increased

Bone Marrow

■ Normal hemosiderin
■ Basophilic stippling in normoblasts

Chemistries

■ Increased free erythrocyte protoporphyrin
■ Normal serum ferritin level
■ Increased λ-aminolevulinic acid levels
■ Normal porphobilinogen
■ Increased blood lead levels

Diagnostic Scheme

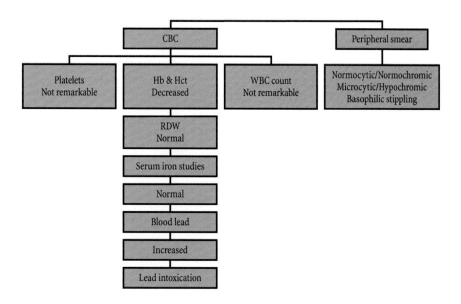

SIDEROBLASTIC ANEMIA

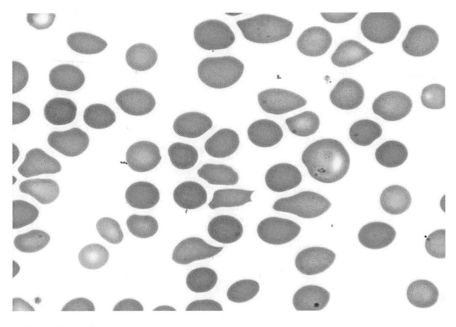

Figure IIA2-19   Peripheral blood smear.

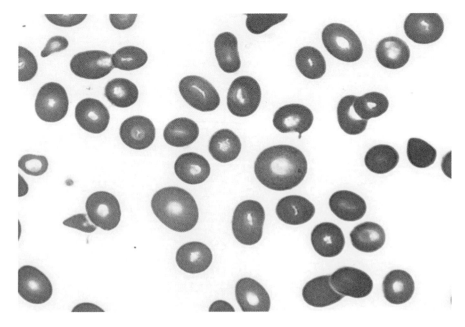

Figure IIA2-20   Peripheral blood smear.

Clinical Features

- Hepatosplenomegaly
- Two classifications:
  - Inherited
    - Usually sex linked
    - May be autosomal
  - Acquired
    - Idiopathic (a type of myelodysplastic syndrome—refractory anemia with ringed sideroblasts [RARS])
    - Secondary (e.g., drugs)

Pathology

- Common features
  - Ineffective erythropoiesis
  - Increased levels of tissue iron (ringed sideroblasts)
  - Failure of protoporphyrin and heme synthesis due to abnormal enzyme activity
- Inherited
  - Symptoms appear early owing to abnormal heme synthesis enzymes
- Idiopathic
  - Clonal disorder
  - Abnormal red blood cell distribution
  - Abnormal heme synthesis enzymes
- Secondary
  - Drugs
    - Inhibition of enzymes

Laboratory Features

White Blood Cells

- Normal to decreased

Platelets

- Not remarkable

Red Blood Cells

- Commonly microcytic/hypochromic anemia
- Dimorphism
- Increased red blood cell distribution width
- Reticulocyte count normal or slightly increased
- Basophilic stippling
- Pappenheimer bodies

Bone Marrow

- Erythroid hyperplasia
- Large numbers of sideroblasts and ringed sideroblasts

Chemistries

- Increased hemosiderin
- Increased serum iron
- Normal or decreased total iron binding capacity
- Normal or increased % saturation
- Increased serum ferritin level

Diagnostic Scheme

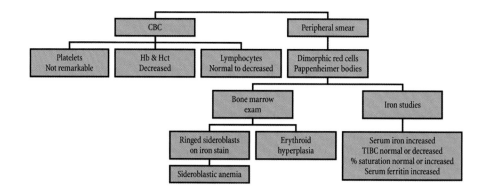

Megaloblastic Anemias

FOLIC ACID DEFICIENCY

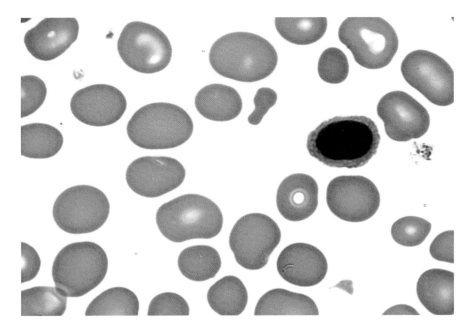

Figure **IIA3-1**   Peripheral blood smear.

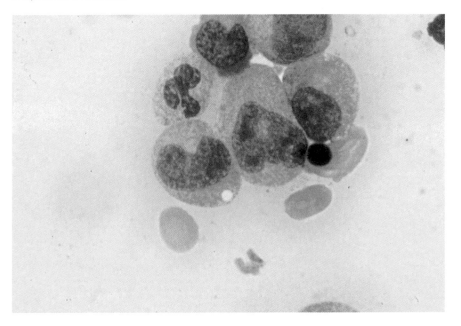

Figure **IIA3-2**   Bone marrow smear.

Clinical Features

- Usually affects the hematopoietic and gastrointestinal systems
- Neurologic system is *not* affected
- Anemia onset may occur 2–3 months after deficiency and may be severe
- Splenomegaly may be present
- History of food faddism, alcoholism, or poor dietary intake
- Glossitis

Pathology

- Defective DNA synthesis due to folate deficiency
  - Ineffective hematopoiesis
  - Dietary deficiency—levels can decrease within 1 month of deficient intake
  - Increased demands—pregnancy
  - Malabsorption
    - Nontropical sprue (gluten-sensitive enteropathy)
    - Tropical sprue
  - Drug therapy
    - Phenytoin
    - Methotrexate

Laboratory Features

White Blood Cells

- Granulocytopenia
- Hypersegmented neutrophils

Platelets

- Thrombocytopenia

Red Blood Cells

- Macrocytic, normochromic anemia
- Presence of macroovalocytes
- Presence of nucleated red blood cells
- Howell-Jolly bodies, Cabot rings, basophilic stippling
- Reticulocyte count normal or decreased
- No polychromasia
- Red blood cell distribution width increased

Bone Marrow

- Megaloblastic erythroid precursors
- Giant myelocytes and metamyelocytes may be seen
- Megakaryocytes may exhibit hyperlobulation and are increased in number

Chemistries

- Indirect bilirubin level increased
- Serum lactic dehydrogenase level increased
- Serum folate level decreased
- Red blood cell folate level decreased
- Methylmalonic acid level normal
- Serum B_{12} level normal or decreased
- Homocysteine level increased

Diagnostic Scheme

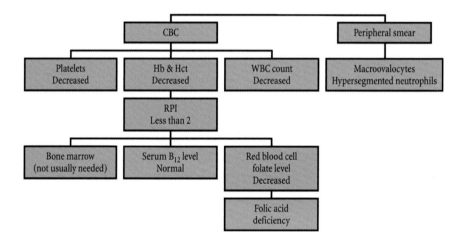

VITAMIN B$_{12}$ DEFICIENCY (PERNICIOUS ANEMIA)

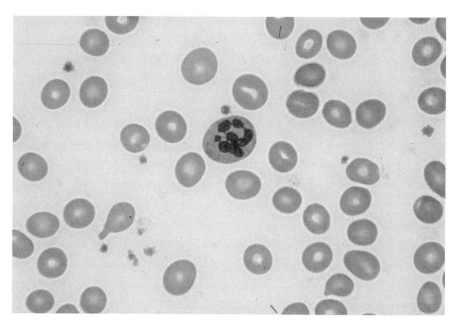

Figure IIA3-3   Peripheral blood smear.

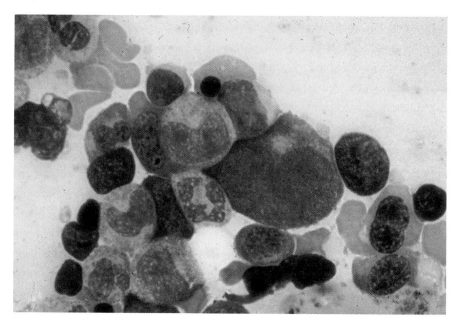

Figure IIA3-4   Bone marrow smear.

Clinical Features

- Usually occurs in persons older than 60 years
- Insidious onset
- Fatigue, weakness, yellowish waxy pallor
- Smooth tongue
- Gastrointestinal complaints
- Paresthesia, mental changes, spastic gait

Pathology

- Abnormal DNA synthesis
  - Ineffective hematopoiesis
- Causes
  - Dietary lack of vitamin B_{12} (rare in the United States)
  - Antibodies to intrinsic factor or antibodies to the parietal cell components
  - Decreased ileal absorption
  - Decreased availability (anatomic abnormalities)
  - Transcobalamin II deficiency
  - Cellular metabolic disorders (nitrous oxide)

Laboratory Features

White Blood Cells

- Neutropenia
- Hypersegmented neutrophils and eosinophils

Platelets

- Thrombocytopenia
- Large platelets present

Red Blood Cells

- Macrocytic, normochromic anemia
- Oval macrocytes
- Anisocytosis, poikilocytosis
- Nucleated red blood cells on peripheral smear
- Howell-Jolly bodies, basophilic stippling, Cabot rings
- Reticulocyte relative number normal but reticulocyte production index <2

Bone Marrow

■ Hypercellular, myeloid:erythroid ratio about 1:1
■ Megaloblastic in erythroid granulocytic and megakaryocytic cell lines
■ Giant metamyelocytes present

Chemistries

■ Increased lactic dehydrogenase level
■ Increased unconjugated bilirubin level
■ Decreased haptoglobin level
■ Increased iron level
■ Decreased B_{12} levels

Diagnostic Scheme

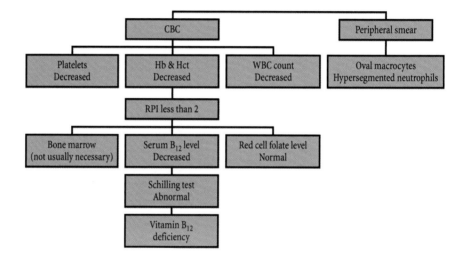

CHAPTER

4

Hypoproliferative Anemias

ANEMIA CAUSED BY MYELOPHTHISIS

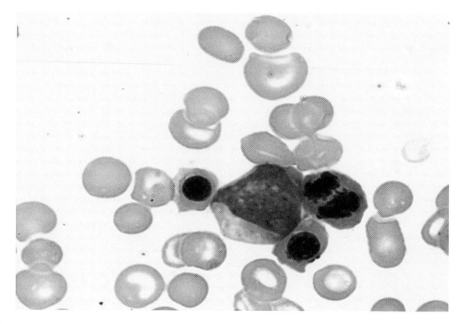

Figure IIA4-1   Peripheral blood smear.

Clinical Features

- Weakness, fatigue
- Hepatosplenomegaly
- Hypersplenism

Pathology

- Marrow invasion (myelophthisis)
  - Tumor
  - Infection
  - Myeloproliferative disorders
  - Other hematologic disorders

Laboratory Features

White Blood Cells

- Variable
- Immature granulocytes seen on the peripheral smear

Platelets

- Occasional giant platelets
- Normal to decreased

Red Blood Cells

- Normocytic, normochromic
- Poikilocytosis
- Fragmented cells
- Dacryocytes
- Nucleated red blood cells seen on the peripheral smear

Bone Marrow

- Nonspecific changes or even normal morphology
- Bone marrow biopsy may reveal fibrosis

Diagnostic Scheme

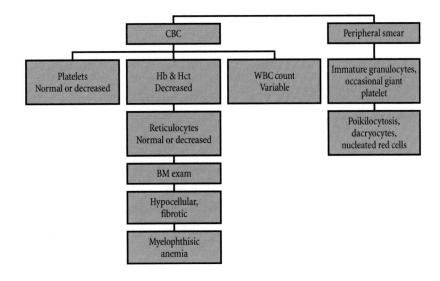

ACQUIRED APLASTIC ANEMIA

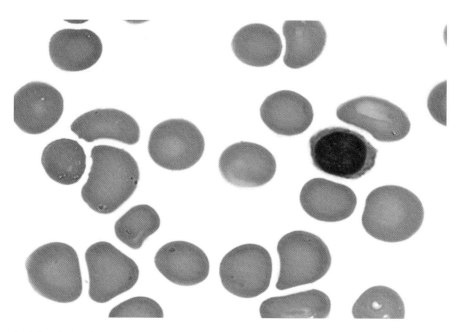

Figure **IIA4-2**   Peripheral blood smear.

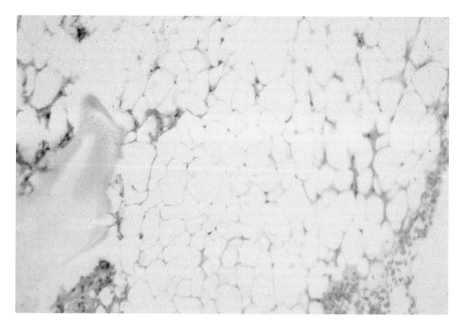

Figure **IIA4-3**   Bone marrow biopsy.

Clinical Features

- Weakness
- Dizziness
- Increased tendency for bruising
- Infections

Pathology

- Pancytopenia
  - Idiopathic
  - Chemical agents
  - Antimicrobials
  - Immunologic disorders
  - Radiation
  - Viral infections
- Decreased CD34 stem cells
- Paroxysmal nocturnal hemoglobinuria may develop in about one-quarter of cases

Laboratory Features

White Blood Cells

- Decreased neutrophils
- Lymphocyte count is normal

Platelets

- Decreased

Red Blood Cells

- Normocytic, normochromic anemia but may be slightly macrocytic
- Red blood cell distribution width normal
- Corrected reticulocyte count decreased

Bone Marrow

- Hypocellular

Criteria for the Diagnosis of Severe Aplastic Anemia

- Neutrophil count less than 0.5×10^9/L
- Platelet count $<20 \times 10^9$/L
- Corrected reticulocyte count $<1\%$ of red blood cells
- Bone marrow cellularity $<30\%$
- No other pathology

Diagnostic Scheme

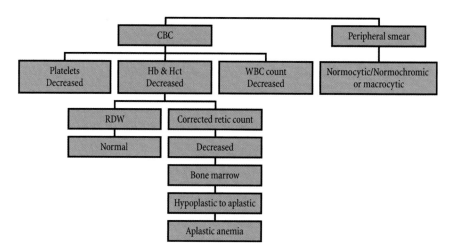

CONGENITAL DYSERYTHROPOIETIC ANEMIA

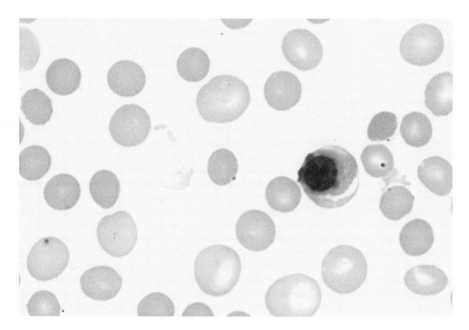

Figure **IIA4-4**   Peripheral blood smear.

Clinical Features

- Type I
  - Autosomal recessive inheritance
  - Male:female ratio 1.25:1
  - Icterus, splenomegaly , brown skin pigmentation, finger and toe abnormalities
- Type II
  - Autosomal recessive inheritance
  - Male:female ratio 1:1
  - Jaundice, hepatosplenomegaly, gallstones
- Type III
  - Autosomal dominance inheritance
  - Male:female ratio 1.9:1

Pathology

- Abnormal erythroid production
- Inherited marrow disorders
- Ineffective erythropoiesis because a discrepancy exists between erythroid output from marrow to circulation, resulting in anemia

Laboratory Features

Type I

White Blood Cells

- Not remarkable

Platelets

- Not remarkable

Red Blood Cells

- Mild anemia
- Reticulocyte count 1–7% of red blood cells
- Mean corpuscular volume slightly increased
- Anisocytosis, poikilocytosis
- Basophilic stippling
- Acidified serum test result negative

Bone Marrow

- Erythroid hyperplasia
- Megaloblastic
- Chromatin bridging

Type II

White Blood Cells

- Not remarkable

Platelets

- Not remarkable

Red Blood Cells

- Normocytic/normochromic anemia
- Anisocytosis, poikilocytosis
- Dacryocytes
- Basophilic stippling
- Cells lysed by 30% acidified sera from healthy persons but not by the patient's own serum
- Negative sugar water test result

Bone Marrow

- Gaucher-like cells
- Erythroid hyperplasia
- Not megaloblastic
- Binuclearity, multinuclearity

Type III

White Blood Cells

- Not remarkable

Platelets

- Not remarkable

Red Blood Cells

- Mild to moderate anemia
- Mean corpuscular volume normal to slightly increased
- Negative acidified serum test result

Bone Marrow

- Erythroid hyperplasia
- Not megaloblastic
- Multinuclearity

Diagnostic Scheme

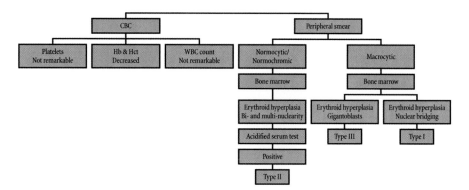

CONGENITAL PURE RED BLOOD CELL APLASIA (DIAMOND-BLACKFAN ANEMIA)

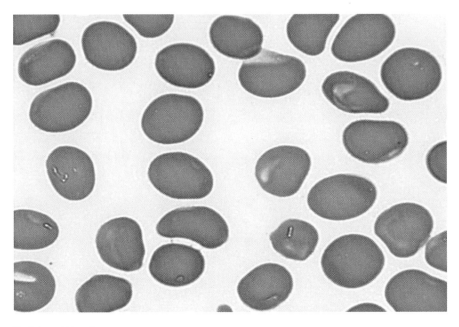

Figure IIA4-5   Peripheral blood smear.

Clinical Features

- Congenital anomalies of kidneys, eyes, skeleton, and heart
- Pallor, listlessness, poor appetite, and failure to thrive, which may progress to congestive heart failure with breathlessness
- Hepatosplenomegaly

Pathology

- Etiology basically unknown
- Intrinsic defect of erythroid precursors—may be a deficiency of adenosine deaminase and purine nucleoside phosphorylase
- The decreased purine nucleoside phosphorylase may result in the accumulation of toxic metabolites that inhibit cell replication
- Red blood cell precursors are not responsive to erythropoietin

Laboratory Features

White Blood Cells

■ Normal to slightly decreased

Platelets

■ Normal to slightly increased

Red Blood Cells

■ Decreased
■ Reticulocyte count decreased
■ Erythropoietin increased

Bone Marrow

■ Myeloid elements appear normal
■ Erythroid precursors decreased with a predominance of pronormoblasts

Chemistries

■ Serum iron level normal to slightly increased
■ % iron saturation increased

Diagnostic Scheme

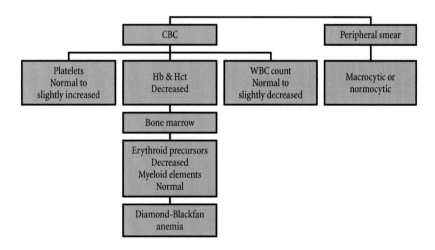

FANCONI'S ANEMIA

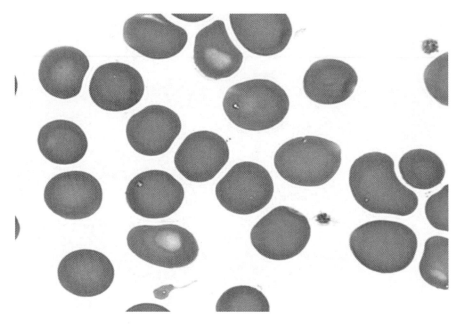

Figure IIA4-6   Peripheral blood smear.

Clinical Features

- Short stature
- Skin pigmentation
- Renal anomalies
- Bone dysplasia
- Microcephaly
- Mental retardation
- Infections
- Male:female ratio 1-3:1

Pathology

- Autosomal recessive inheritance
- Underlying defect is not entirely elucidated, may be a defect in DNA repair
- Chromosomal abnormalities include breaks, gaps, endoreplications, rearrangements, and exchanges

Laboratory Features

White Blood Cells

- Decreased granulocytes

Platelets

- Decreased

Red Blood Cells

- Macrocytic anemia
- Increased hemoglobin F

Bone Marrow

- Hypocellular
- Possible dyserythropoiesis

Diagnostic Scheme

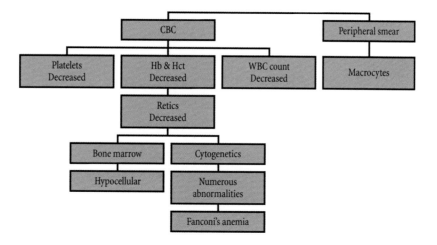

PURE RED CELL APLASIA

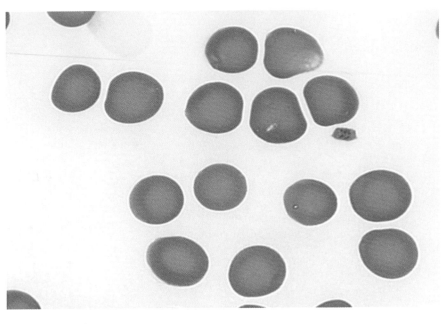

Figure IIA4-7   Peripheral blood smear.

Clinical Features

- Severe anemia—weakness, headache, vertigo, fatigue, tinnitus, and irritability
- Primary
  - Idiopathic
  - Immune mediated
- Secondary
  - Associated with thymoma
  - Neoplasia
  - Drugs
  - Infections

Pathology

- Erythropoiesis inhibited primarily by immune mechanism
- T cells, particularly large granular lymphocytes, may be involved in the suppression of erythropoiesis
- Specific attachment on erythroid precursors by the parvo virus B-19
- Clonal abnormality as a prodrome to myelodysplastic syndrome

Laboratory Features

White Blood Cells

■ Not remarkable

Platelets

■ Not remarkable

Red Blood Cells

■ Normocytic/normochromic anemia
■ Hemoglobin level decreased
■ Hematocrit level decreased
■ Reticulocytes absent

Bone Marrow

■ Absence of erythroid cells
■ Myeloid and megakaryocytic elements are preserved

Diagnostic Scheme

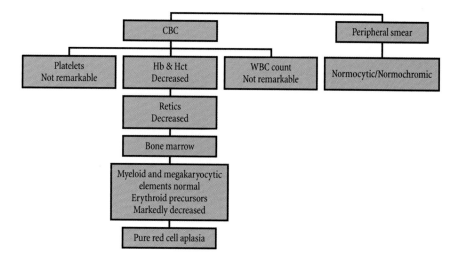

CHAPTER

5

Qualitative Hemoglobinopathies

HEMOGLOBIN C

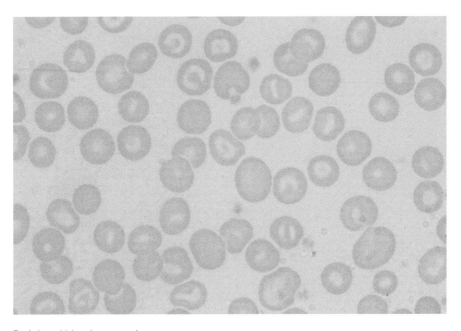

Figure IIA5-1   Peripheral blood smear—heterozygous.

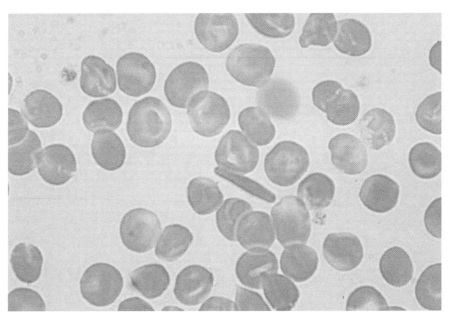

Figure IIA5-2   Peripheral blood smear—homozygous.

Clinical Features

- Mild to moderate hemolysis
- Palpable splenomegaly
- Cholelithiasis and aplastic crises may occur
- Arthralgia is common
- May be abdominal pain
- Hemoglobin C trait has no clinical manifestations

Pathology

- α_2/β_2 (glutamic acid replaced by lysine on amino acid 6)
- Relative insolubility of hemoglobin C causes red blood cells to become rigid
- Loss of potassium and cell hydration
- Cell is subject to fragmentation and loss of membrane material, resulting in microspherocytes

Laboratory Features

White Blood Cells

- Not remarkable

Platelets

- Not remarkable

Red Blood Cells

- Microspherocytes present
- Reticulocyte count 4–8%
- Hematocrit level approximately 0.25-0.37 L/L
- Approximately 30–100% target cells
- C crystals seen in oxyhemoglobin state

Hemoglobin Electrophoresis

- Homozygous: about 100% hemoglobin C
- Heterozygous: 30–40% C, 50–60% A, slight increase in A_2

Diagnostic Scheme

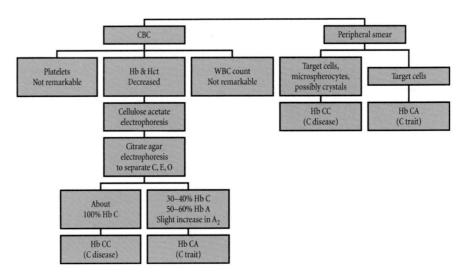

HEMOGLOBIN D

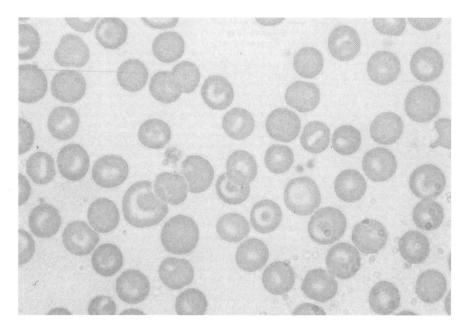

Figure IIA5-3   Peripheral blood smear.

Clinical Features

- Disorder is rare
- Homozygous individuals may have a mild anemia
- Both homozygous and heterozygous individuals are asymptomatic

Pathology

- α/β_2 (glutamic acid replaced by glycine on amino acid 121)
- Many variants are found
  - Hemoglobin D-Punjab and hemoglobin D Los Angeles are the most commonly encountered of the D hemoglobins in American Blacks (0.02%)

Laboratory Features

White Blood Cells

■ Not remarkable

Platelets

■ Not remarkable

Red Blood Cells

■ Homozygotes may have a normal hemoglobin level and no evidence of hemolysis
■ Indices normal
■ May see target cells
■ May see decreased osmotic fragility

Hemoglobin Electrophoresis

■ Homozygous
 ■ 95% D and normal A_2
 ■ Hemoglobin D migrates with S at pH 8.6 but does not sickle
 ■ Hemoglobin D migrates with A on acid electrophoresis

Diagnostic Scheme

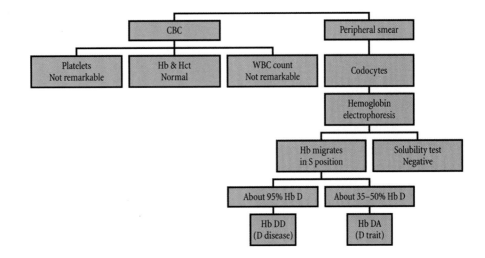

HEMOGLOBIN E

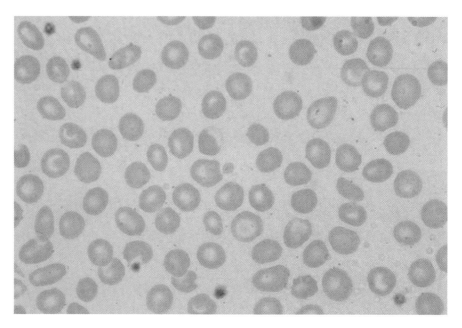

Figure IIA5-4   Peripheral blood smear.

Clinical Features

- Homozygous: mild or asymptomatic, microcytic anemia with decreased erythrocyte survival
- Heterozygous: symptomless, microcytosis

Pathology

- Substitution of lysine for glutamic acid in the β chain
- Hemoglobin is slightly unstable with oxidant stress
- Oxygen dissociation curve is shifted to the right, indicating that hemoglobin E has decreased oxygen affinity

Laboratory Features

White Blood Cells

■ Not remarkable

Platelets

■ Not remarkable

Red Blood Cells

■ Hemoglobin level is 12.0–13.0 g/dL
■ Decreased mean corpuscular volume
■ Target cells present
■ Increased red blood cells
■ Normal or decreased reticulocyte count

Hemoglobin Electrophoresis

■ Presence of hemoglobin E

Diagnostic Scheme

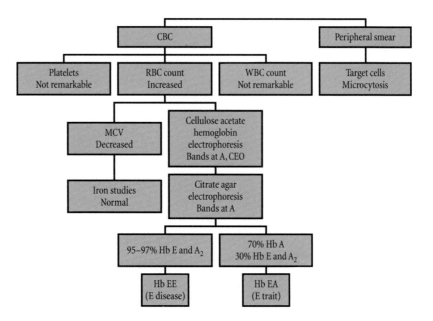

HEMOGLOBIN E/β THALASSEMIA

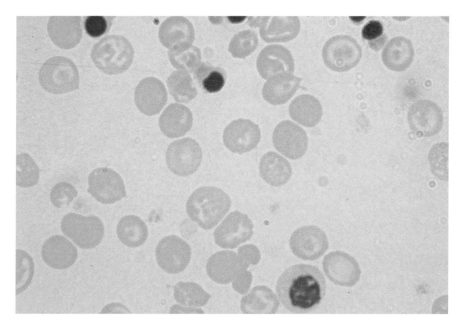

Figure IIA5-5   Peripheral blood smear.

Clinical Features

- Moderate to severe anemia
- The most severe type is E/β^0
- Anemia is generally more severe than in patients with hemoglobin S/β
- Anemia is more severe than in E trait
- Splenomegaly

Pathology

- This is the most common combination in Southeast Asians
- Double heterozygous for hemoglobin E and β thalassemia

Laboratory Features

White Blood Cells

■ Not remarkable

Platelets

■ Not remarkable

Red Blood Cells

■ Decreased hemoglobin and hematocrit levels
■ Microcytic, hypochromic anemia
■ Presence of nucleated red blood cells

Hemoglobin Electrophoresis (Cellulose Acetate, pH 8.4)

■ Bands at A, F, CEO

Diagnostic Scheme

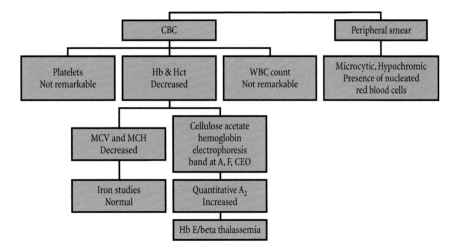

HEMOGLOBIN S

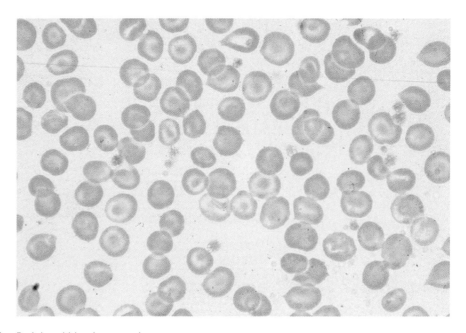

Figure IIA5-6   Peripheral blood smear—heterozygous.

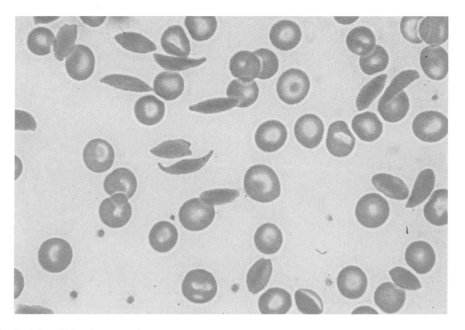

Figure IIA5-7   Peripheral blood smear—homozygous.

Clinical Features

- Homozygous
  - A disease state that occurs in approximately 0.3–1.3% of American Blacks
  - Person with this disorder may present with fever, effusion of joints, bone deformities, loss of renal function, priapism , enlarged liver, ocular manifestations, leg ulcers, frequent infections, decreased spleen function, complications during pregnancy, and/or cerebrovascular accidents
  - Acute episodes may be manifest
- Heterozygous
  - The individual possesses one normal beta gene and one S gene
  - In American Blacks, the frequency is approximately 8%
  - No clinical symptoms are associated with the trait, but episodes of hematuria may occur

Pathology

- A single nucleotide base change in the codon responsible for the synthesis of the sixth amino acid in the β-globulin chain, resulting in the substitution of valine for glutamic acid
- The deoxyhemoglobin polymerizes within the red blood cell
- Extravascular hemolysis of sickled cells takes place, causing a chronic hemolytic anemia

Laboratory Features

Homozygous

White Blood Cells

- Usually increased during a crisis, may be up to $25 \times 10^9/L$

Platelets

- Normal to increased

Red Blood Cells

- Normocytic/normochromic anemia
- Hemoglobin level 6.5–10.0 g/dL
- Reticulocyte count is increased (10–20%)
- Red blood cell distribution width is increased
- Smear shows polychromasia, codocytes, Howell-Jolly bodies, nucleated red blood cells, and drepanocytes

Bone Marrow

- Erythroid hyperplasia caused by chronic hemolysis

Hemoglobin Electrophoresis

- 0% hemoglobin A
- 80–99% hemoglobin S
- Slightly increased hemoglobin A_2
- 1–20% hemoglobin F

Heterozygous

White Blood Cells

- Not remarkable

Platelets

- Not remarkable

Red Blood Cells

- Codocytes
- Hemoglobin and hematocrit levels normal

Bone Marrow

- Not remarkable

Hemoglobin Electrophoresis

- 50–65% hemoglobin A
- 35–45% hemoglobin S
- Normal to slightly increased hemoglobin A_2
- Normal hemoglobin F

Diagnostic Scheme

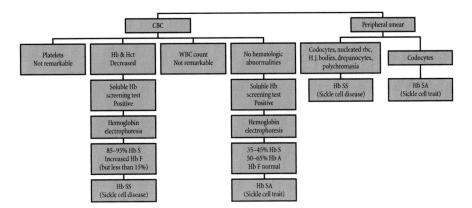

HEMOGLOBIN S/β THALASSEMIA

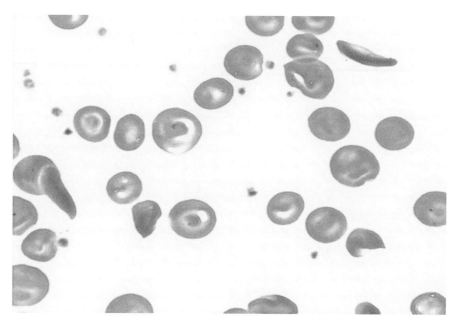

Figure IIA5-8   Peripheral blood smear.

Clinical Features

- S/β^0—severity comparable to that seen in sickle cell anemia
- S/β^+—milder clinical course comparable to SC disease
- Splenomegaly

Pathology

- β thalassemia gene reduces the rate of synthesis of beta^A chain, resulting in a predominance of beta^S

Laboratory Features

White Blood Cells

- Not remarkable

Platelets

■ Not remarkable

Red Blood Cells

■ Microcytic/hypochromic anemia
■ Decreased mean corpuscular volume

Hemoglobin Electrophoresis

■ S/β^0—mostly hemoglobin S, increased A_2, variable F and no A
■ S/β^+—hemoglobin S about 11%, A_2 about 6%

Hemoglobin S/C Disease

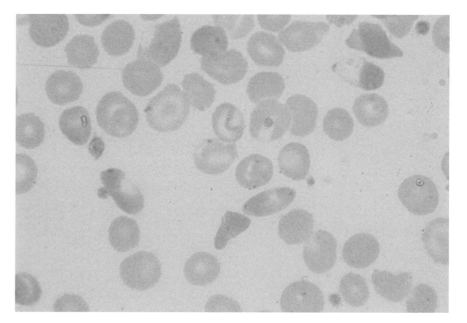

Figure IIA5-9   Peripheral blood smear.

Clinical Features

■ Splenomegaly
■ Proliferative retinopathy
■ Aseptic necrosis of long bones
■ Muscle, bone, and joint pain
■ Hematuria
■ Acute pulmonary disease
■ Splenic infarction
■ Vaso-occlusive crisis during pregnancy, surgery, or medical emergency

Pathology

■ Both β chains are abnormal
■ Less frequent and less severe than sickle cell anemia
■ More severe than sickle trait of C trait

Laboratory Features

White Blood Cells

■ Not remarkable

Platelets

■ Not remarkable

Red Blood Cells

■ Knizocytes, stomatocytes, and target cells present
■ Increased mean corpuscular hemoglobin
■ Microcytic anemia
■ Sickling not prominent
■ SC crystals

Bone Marrow

■ Normoblastic hyperplasia

Hemoglobin Electrophoresis

■ Equal amounts of hemoglobin S and hemoglobin C
■ 1–2% hemoglobin F
■ Trace of A_2

Diagnostic Scheme

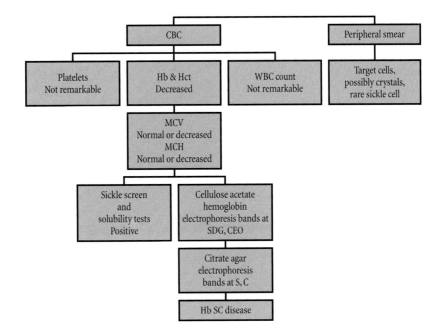

UNSTABLE HEMOGLOBINS

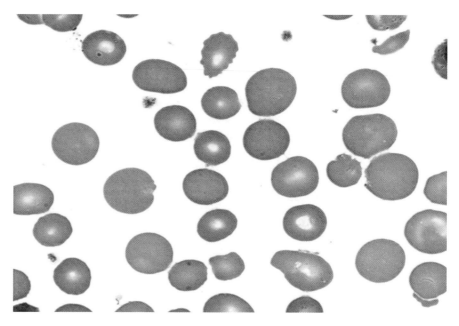

Figure IIA5-10   Peripheral blood smear.

Clinical Features

- Hemoglobin denaturation and hemolysis may occur spontaneously
- Symptoms may occur only after drug administration, infection, or other changes to the normal environment
- Jaundice and splenomegaly occur because of increased red blood cell hemolysis
- Excretion of dark urine
- Cyanosis may result from the formation of sulfhemoglobin
- Methemoglobin

Pathology

- Amino acid substitutions in critical internal portions of the globin chains
- Abnormal hemoglobin precipitates as Heinz bodies, which attach to the inner surface of the membrane and can cause cell rigidity, membrane damage, and, thus, erythrocyte hemolysis
- Homozygous state is incompatible with life
- Oxygen stability may be increased or decreased depending on where the amino acid substitution is located
- Hemoglobin with high oxygen affinity is usually accompanied by erythrocytosis
  - Oxygen dissociation curve is shifted to the left
  - Decreased amount of oxygen released to the tissues and increased erythropoietin levels
- Hemoglobin with decreased oxygen affinity may be asymptomatic
  - Oxygen dissociation curve is shifted to the right
  - Increased amount of oxygen delivered to the tissues

Laboratory Features

White Blood Cells

- Not remarkable

Platelets

- Not remarkable

Red Blood Cells

- Normochromic/normocytic anemia
- Slight decrease in mean corpuscular hemoglobin and mean corpuscular hemoglobin concentration
- Reticulocyte count is increased
- Basophilic stippling, bite cells, and small contracted cells may be present
- Osmotic fragility abnormal after 24-hour incubation
- Heat instability test result is positive
- Isopropanol stability test result is positive
- Hemoglobin electrophoresis is abnormal in about 45% of cases—A_2 and F are sometimes increased
- Heinz bodies are seen on brilliant cresyl blue stain

Diagnostic Scheme

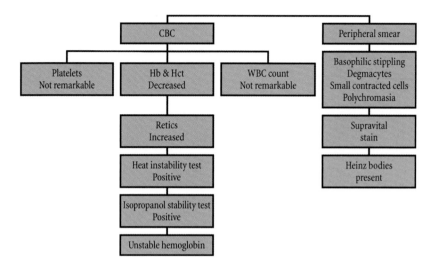

CHAPTER

6

Hemolytic Anemias

COLD AGGLUTININ DISEASE

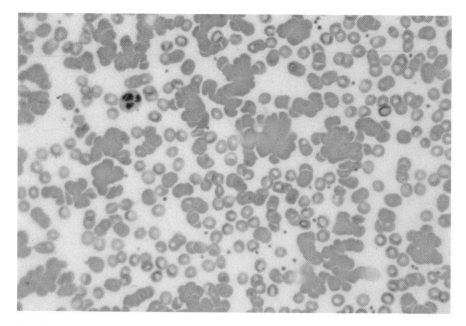

Figure IIA6-1   Peripheral blood smear.

Clinical Features

- Peak incidence in patients older than 50 years
- Onset may be sudden and severe, but the syndrome usually does not last >1–3 weeks
- In adults, the anemia is usually gradual and not as severe as in children
- Purplish discoloration of fingers, toes, nose, ears, or other peripheral areas that are exposed to cold
- Numbness of extremities when exposed to cold
- Splenomegaly

Pathology

- Can be secondary in patients with lymphoproliferative diseases, infectious mononucleosis, or *Mycoplasma pneumoniae* infections
- Patients may develop antibodies directed against the I or i antigens on red blood cells
- Usually an IgM antibody that activates complement and hemolysis results
- In children and young adults, the syndrome is brought on by viral infections
- Diminished erythropoiesis caused by the infection

Laboratory Features

White Blood Cells

■ Normal or falsely elevated

Platelets

■ Not remarkable

Red Blood Cells

■ Mean corpuscular volume increased when blood cools to room temperature
■ Reticulocyte count increased
■ Agglutination rouleaux
■ Mild to moderate anisocytosis, poikilocytosis
■ Polychromatophilia
■ Falsely decreased red blood cell count
■ Mean corpuscular hemoglobin concentration falsely increased due to falsely decreased hematocrit levels

Bone Marrow

■ Erythroid hyperplasia

Serological Tests

■ Direct antihuman globulin test (DAT) positive, with polyspecific antisera and anti-C3d
■ Cold agglutinin titer of ≥1000 in saline at 4°C.

Diagnostic Scheme

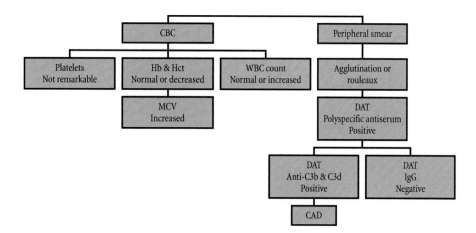

GLUCOSE-6-PHOSPHATE DEHYDROGENASE DEFICIENCY

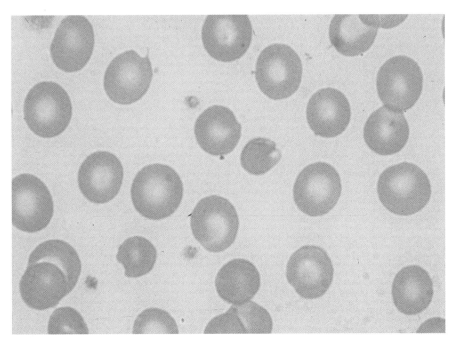

Peripheral blood smear.

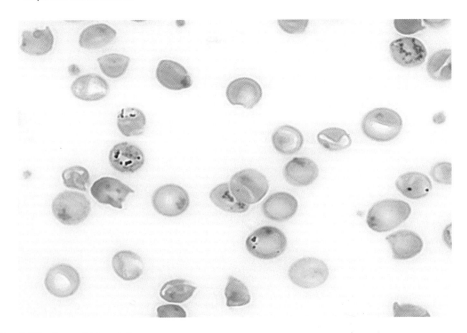

Brilliant cresyl blue stain.

Clinical Features

- No clinical symptoms unless exposed to chemicals or drug oxidants or severe infections
- Chronic hemolysis
- Jaundice is not prominent
- Abdominal and low back pain
- Urine is dark or black because of hemoglobinuria
- Classification is based on degree of hemolysis and enzyme deficiency
- Classes I, II, and III are clinically significant

Pathology

- The glucose-6-phosphate dehydrogenase gene is located on the X chromosome
- Red blood cells deficient in glucose-6-phosphate dehydrogenase are susceptible to oxidation and hemolysis
- Nicotinamide adenine dinucleotide phosphate production is impaired
- Build up of cellular oxidants leads to erythrocyte injury and hemolysis
- Hemoglobin is oxidized to methemoglobin, which precipitates in the form of Heinz bodies
- Heinz bodies attach to the red blood cell membrane, causing increased permeability to cations, osmotic fragility, and cell rigidity
- Red blood cells have a rigid cell wall, with the hemoglobin confined to one part of the cytosol

Laboratory Features

White Blood Cells

- Increased during attacks

Platelets

- Normal

Red Blood Cells

- Normocytic/normochromic anemia
- Increased reticulocyte count after hemolytic crises
- Heinz bodies
- Polychromasia
- Occasional spherocytes
- Degmacytes
- Positive fluorescent screening test result for glucose-6-phosphate dehydrogenase deficiency

- Quantitative direct enzyme assay for glucose-6-phosphate dehydrogenase decreased
- Positive Heinz body test result

Chemistries

- Indirect bilirubin and lactic dehydrogenase levels may be increased
- Haptoglobin level decreased during attacks

Diagnostic Scheme

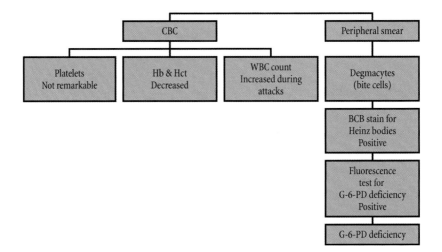

HEREDITARY ACANTHOCYTOSIS

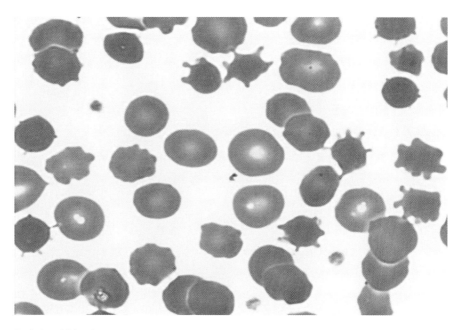

Figure **IIA6-4**

Peripheral blood smear.

Clinical Features

- Autosomal recessive disease
- Major symptoms due to vitamin E deficiency
- Malabsorption of fat, retinitis pigmentosa, neurologic damage, mental retardation, and delayed growth development

Pathology

- Deficiency in apoprotein
- Defect in beta lipoprotein particle assembly and secretion in the intestine and liver
- Deficient absorption and transport of fat-soluble vitamins A, D, E, and K
- Red blood cells have an increased sphingomyelin:lecithin ratio that leads to acanthocytosis
- Deficiency in triglyceride microsomal transfer protein, which is necessary for the assembly and secretion of apolipoprotein B–containing lipoproteins from the liver and intestine

Laboratory Features

White Blood Cells

- Not remarkable

Platelets

- Not remarkable

Red Blood Cells

- Mild normocytic/normochromic anemia
- Indices normal
- Reticulocyte count normal or slightly increased
- Acanthocytes
- Increased osmotic fragility

Chemistries

- Triglycerides decreased
- Cholesterol level usually <50 mg/dL
- Low-density lipoprotein, very low-density lipoprotein, chylomicrons decreased

Diagnostic Scheme

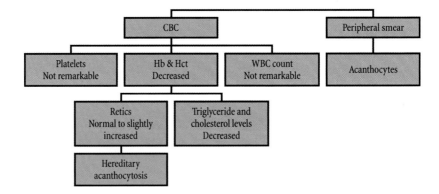

HEREDITARY ELLIPTOCYTOSIS

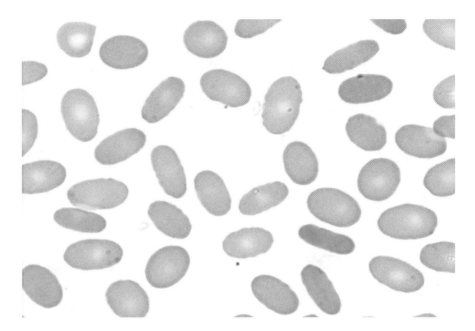

Figure **IIA6-5**   Peripheral blood smear—common hereditary elliptocytosis.

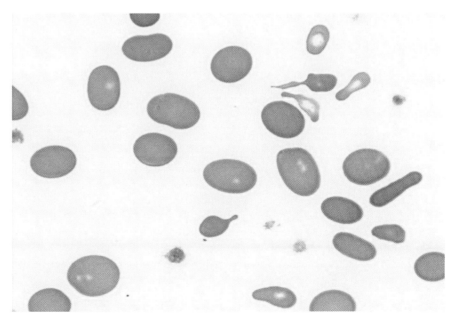

Figure **IIA6-6**   Peripheral blood smear—hereditary pyropoikilocytosis.

Clinical Features

- About 90% of patients show no overt signs of hemolysis
- Hemolysis is usually mild and well compensated by the bone marrow
- Morphologic classification
  - Common hereditary elliptocytosis
    - Inherited as an autosomal dominant trait
    - Ranges from asymptomatic to severe clinical disease
  - Spherocytic hereditary elliptocytosis
    - Inherited as an autosomal dominant trait
    - Presence of hemolysis
  - Stomatocytic hereditary elliptocytosis (Melanesian or Southeast Asian ovalocytosis)
    - Inherited as a recessive trait
    - Occurs in about 0.2–0.5%
    - Mild or absent hemolytic component
    - Cation permeability increased
  - Hereditary pyropoikilocytosis
    - Inherited as a recessive trait
    - Presents in infancy or early childhood
    - Microspherocytes
    - Severe red blood cell fragmentation and hemolysis
    - Hyperbilirubinemia may require exchange transfusion or phototherapy

Pathology

- The defect is in one of the skeletal proteins in the membrane, which is acquired in the circulation (horizontal membrane protein interaction)
  - Decreased associate of spectrin dimers to form tetramers due to defective spectrin chains
  - Deficient or defective band 4.1, which aids in binding spectrin to actin .
  - Abnormalities of integral proteins (glycophorin C and band 3)
- Membrane fragmentation causes a decrease in cell surface and reduced cell deformability and thus a shortened life span
- Abnormal permeability to sodium and thus increased demands on adenosine triphosphate availability
- In hereditary pyropoikilocytosis, there is a mutant alpha or beta spectrin that shows severe impairment of spectrin dimer self-association and a partial deficiency of spectrin due to decreased alpha spectrin synthesis or an unstable spectrin deficiency

Laboratory Features

White Blood Cells

- Not remarkable

Platelets

- Not remarkable

Red Blood Cells

- Common hereditary elliptocytosis: mild elliptocytosis (15%) to severe fragmentation and poikilocytes
- Spherocytic hereditary elliptocytosis: morphology between spherocytes and elliptocytes
- Stomatocytic hereditary elliptocytosis: round elliptocytes with slit
- Hereditary pyropoikilocytosis: poikilocytosis, microspherocytes, budding of cells

Diagnostic Scheme

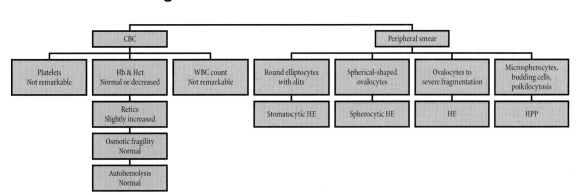

HEREDITARY SPHEROCYTOSIS

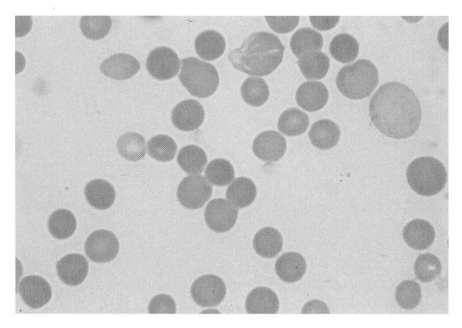

Figure IIA6-7   Peripheral blood smear.

Clinical Features

■ Usually inherited as an autosomal dominant trait, but can be recessive
■ Classically, the patient will have anemia, jaundice, and splenomegaly; however, the symptoms are variable
■ Gallstone formation is not uncommon

Pathology

■ Red blood cell membrane abnormalities
  ■ Spectrin deficiency
  ■ Ankyrin deficiency
  ■ Protein 3 deficiency
  ■ Protein 4.1 deficiency
  ■ Protein 4.2 defect
■ Because of the membrane disorder, microspherocytes are formed that are not deformable and that are sequestered in the spleen
■ A hemolytic anemia may result

Laboratory Features

White Blood Cells

■ Usually normal

Platelets

■ Usually normal

Red Blood Cells

■ Increased mean corpuscular hemoglobin concentration
■ Normal to decreased mean corpuscular volume
■ Normal mean corpuscular hemoglobin
■ Reticulocyte count increased (5–20%)
■ Diffusely basophilic erythrocytes, spherocytes, anisocytosis, and poikilocytosis seen on smear
■ Osmotic fragility increased

Bone Marrow

■ Erythroid hyperplasia

Chemistries

■ Indirect bilirubin level increased
■ Fecal and urine urobilinogen levels increased
■ Lactic dehydrogenase level increased
■ Haptoglobin level decreased

Diagnostic Scheme

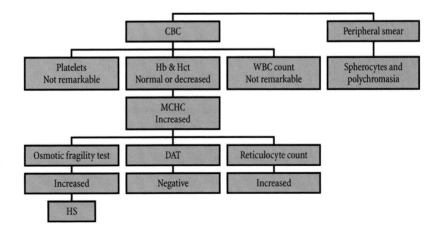

HEREDITARY STOMATOCYTOSIS

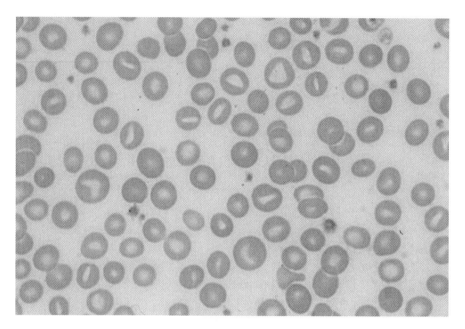

Figure **IIA6-8**   Peripheral blood smear.

Clinical Features

■ On occasion, the patient may have a palpable spleen

Pathology

■ Passive influx of sodium ions exceeds the loss of potassium ions
■ The enzyme sodium-potassium adenosine triphosphatase is overwhelmed and the water content of the cell is increased
■ The surface area:volume ratio is decreased
■ The most common defect is one of the red blood cell membrane protein in the band 7.2b (stomatin)
■ Cells are more avid, which increased thrombotic events

Laboratory Features

White Blood Cells

■ Not remarkable

Platelets

■ Not remarkable

Red Blood Cells

■ Mild to moderate anemia
■ Stomatocytes present
■ Moderate reticulocytosis
■ Increased bilirubin level
■ Osmotic fragility increased
■ Autohemolysis increased

Diagnostic Scheme

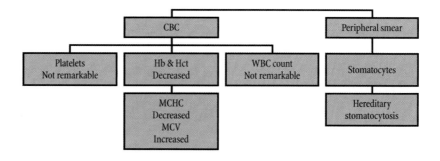

IMMUNE HEMOLYTIC ANEMIA

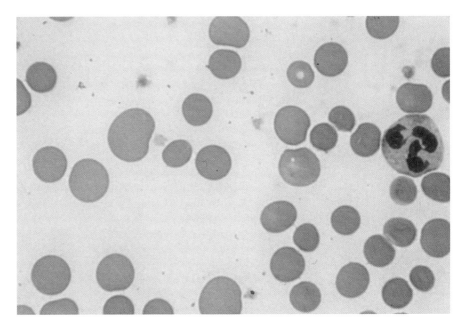

Figure IIA6-9   Peripheral blood smear.

Clinical Features

■ Mild fatigue to dyspnea, syncope, and angina result because of decreased oxygen delivery to tissues
■ Pallor
■ Jaundice

Pathology

■ Destruction of red blood cells by antibodies produced by the patient
■ Destruction of red blood cells by these antibodies is brought about primarily by a mechanism that depends on immune adherence

Laboratory Features

White Blood Cells

- May be elevated due to an increase in neutrophils
- Counts may approach 30×10^9/L

Platelets

- Usually normal

Red Blood Cells

- Hemoglobin and hematocrit levels decreased
- Normocytic/normochromic anemia
- Reticulocyte count increased
- Increased mean corpuscular volume is due to prominent reticulocytosis
- Spherocytes

Bone Marrow

- Hypercellular with erythroid precursors

Diagnostic Scheme

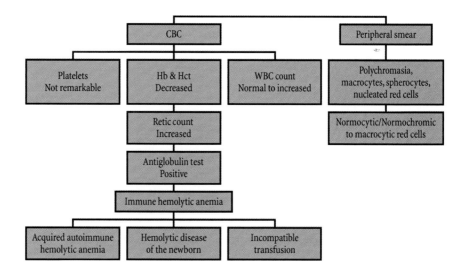

MICROANGIOPATHIC HEMOLYTIC ANEMIA

Figure IIA6-10   Peripheral blood smear.

Clinical Features

- Hemolysis—intravascular
- Thrombotic thrombocytopenic purpura
  - Occurs frequently in young adults
  - Hemorrhage into the tissues
  - Fever
  - Renal dysfunction
  - Neurologic abnormalities
- Hemolytic uremic syndrome
  - Occurs most often in children after viral illnesses
  - Fever
  - Renal failure
  - May show neurologic findings
- Disseminated intravascular coagulation
  - Associated with trauma, massive transfusion, obstetric complications, sepsis, carcinoma, and others
  - Hemorrhagic tendencies
  - Progressive renal dysfunction

Pathology

- Localized intravascular coagulation in which fibrin strands bridge the arteriolar lumen when supplying blood in inflamed or neoplastic tissue
- Fibrin strands lop off fragments of red blood cells whose membranes seal, leaving distorted cells
- In thrombotic thrombocytopenic purpura, small platelet thrombi occlude capillaries and arterioles in a variety of organs

Laboratory Features

White Blood Cells

- Not remarkable

Platelets

- Decreased

Red Blood Cells

- Normocytic/normochromic anemia
- Increased reticulocyte count
- Schistocytes
- Polychromatophilia

Diagnostic Scheme

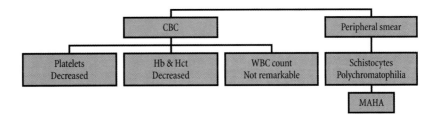

NONIMMUNE HEMOLYTIC ANEMIA

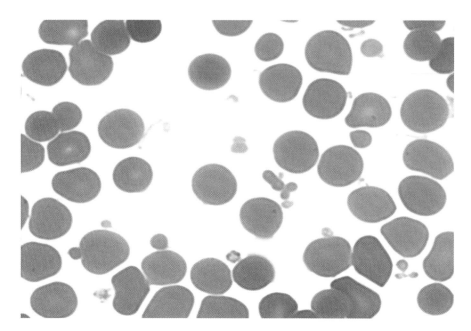

Figure IIA6-11   Peripheral blood smear.

Clinical Features

- Hemolysis—intravascular or extravascular
- Evidence of hemolysis—jaundice, hemoglobinuria, and hemoglobinemia

Pathology

- Thermal injury
  - Red blood cells within the vessels exposed to temperatures above about 50°C are destroyed, causing immediate intravascular fragmentation and lysis
  - Because of increased capillary permeability, plasma is lost from the vessels, resulting in hemoconcentration
- Mechanical injury
  - Red blood cells disintegrate when subjected to strong stretching or shearing forces
  - March hemoglobinuria occurs with prolonged marching or running, and red blood cells are destroyed in the vessels of the feet

Laboratory Features

Thermal Injury

White Blood Cells

- Increased

Platelets

- Not remarkable

Red Blood Cells

- Microspherocytes
- Budding of membrane

Mechanical Injury

White Blood Cells

- Not remarkable

Platelets

- Not remarkable

Red Blood Cells

- Schistocytes
- Keratocytes
- Reticulocyte count increased

Diagnostic Scheme

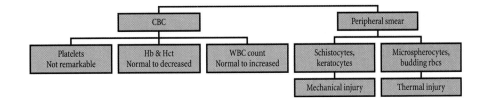

PAROXYSMAL NOCTURNAL HEMOGLOBINURIA

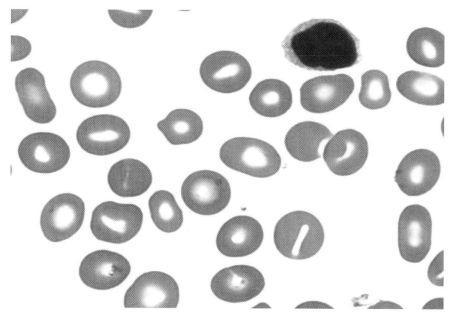

Figure **IIA6-12**   Peripheral blood smear.

Clinical Features

- Rare disorder with severe anemia possible
- Acute episodes of intravascular hemolysis are superimposed on a background of chronic hemolysis
- Hemoglobinuria on voiding after sleep is not a universal finding
- Recurrent venous occlusions may lead to pulmonary embolisms and hepatic and mesenteric vein thrombosis
- May be precipitated by surgery, transfusion, or infections
- Three types of paroxysmal nocturnal hemoglobinuria (PNH) cell may be observed and is associated with the severity of the disease

Pathology

- Somatic mutation in marrow stem cells
- Clonal disorder of hematopoiesis caused by a deficiency of phosphatidylinositol glycan class A
- Abnormal susceptibility to complement-mediated lysis
- The decay-accelerating factor that regulates the activity of C3 convertase is one of the missing proteins

- Loss of surface protein linkage caused by deficiency of glycophosphatidylinositol anchors
- Can progress to acute myelogenous leukemia or myelodysplasia

Laboratory Features

White Blood Cells

- Neutropenia
- Decreased leukocyte alkaline phosphatase (LAP) activity

Platelets

- Thrombocytopenia
- Abnormal platelet function

Red Blood Cells

- Hemolytic anemia
- Iron deficiency may develop with chronic hemolysis
- Acetylcholinesterase activity decreased

Bone Marrow

- Marrow hypoplasia

Immunophenotype

- Decreased CD55, CD59

Chemistries

- Serum haptoglobin level decreased
- Methemalbumin level increased
- Hemoglobinuria
- Hemosiderinuria
- Ham's test result positive
- Sucrose lysis test is the most common screening test

Diagnostic Scheme

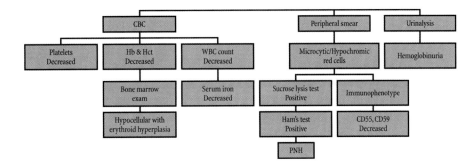

PYRUVATE KINASE DEFICIENCY

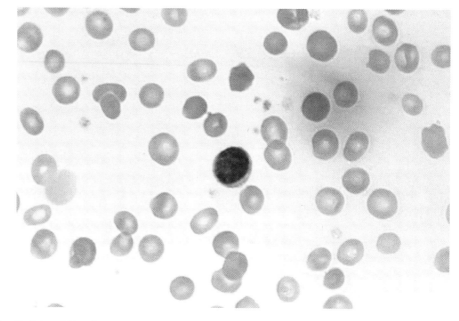

Figure IIA6-13   Peripheral blood smear.

Clinical Features

- Autosomal recessive inheritance
- Most severe types manifest in infancy
- Homozygosity produces clinical disease
- Acquired pyruvate kinase (PK) deficiency has been reported
- Severity ranges from severe neonatal anemia to asymptomatic
- May see splenomegaly, icterus, and gallstones

Pathology

- Most common enzyme deficiency in the Embden-Meyerhof pathway and second most common red blood cell enzyme deficiency
- Adenosine triphosphate levels cannot be maintained at normal levels, and the red blood cell membrane is altered
- Potassium is lost and dehydration results
- Echinocytes are formed and cannot deform in splenic cords—hemolysis results

Laboratory Features

White Blood Cells

- Not remarkable

Platelets

- Not remarkable

Red Blood Cells

- No characteristic cells
- May see echinocytes, macrocytes
- Increased reticulocyte count
- Normocytic/normochromic anemia
- Osmotic fragility normal

Bone Marrow

- Erythroid hyperplasia

Diagnostic Scheme

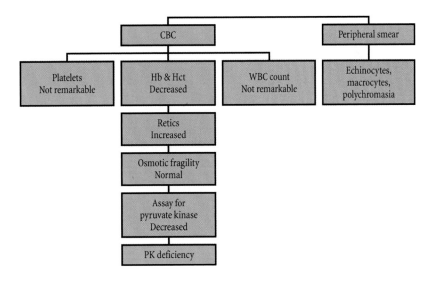

CHAPTER

7

Acute Blood Loss

ANEMIA OF ACUTE BLOOD LOSS

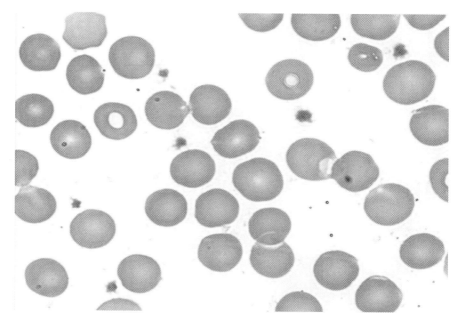

Figure IIA7-1   Peripheral blood smear.

Clinical Features

- Symptoms depend on the amount of blood loss and how fast it was lost
- Lightheadedness, hypotension, and rapid pulse
- Cool, clammy skin
- Unconsciousness and severe shock
- Death

Pathology

- An injury that allows blood to escape from blood vessels into surrounding tissues or outside the body
- If >20% of the total blood volume is lost, oxygen perfusion of tissue is disrupted, resulting in subsequent cell death

Laboratory Features (3–4 hours after the event)

White Blood Cells

■ Increased with shift to the left

Platelets

■ Increased

Red Blood Cells

■ Hemoglobin and hematocrit levels begin to decrease
■ Normocytic/normochromic anemia
■ Increased reticulocytes occur 2–5 days after the event

Bone Marrow

■ Erythroid hyperplasia

Diagnostic Scheme

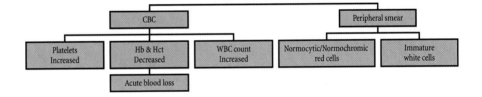

CHAPTER

8

Anemias Associated With Systemic Disorders

CHRONIC RENAL DISEASE

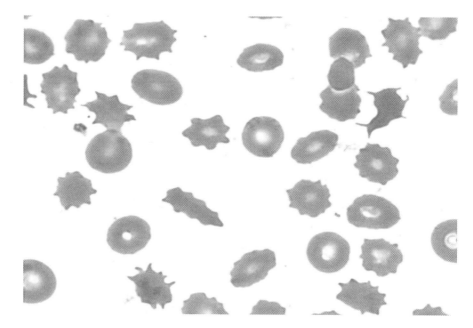

Figure IIA8-1   Peripheral blood smear.

Clinical Features

- Symptoms depend on severity of anemia
- May manifest with gastrointestinal or gynecologic bleeding
- Fatigue

Pathology

- Failure of renal excretory function and accumulation of waste products in plasma causes:
    - Decreased red blood cell survival and mild hemolytic anemia
    - Failure of renal production of erythropoietin
    - Failure of release of erythropoietin

Laboratory Features

White Blood Cells

■ Not remarkable

Platelets

■ Normal to slightly increased
■ Function may be abnormal

Red Blood Cells

■ Normocytic/normochromic anemia
■ Burr cells (echinocytes)
■ Reticulocyte count normal

Diagnostic Scheme

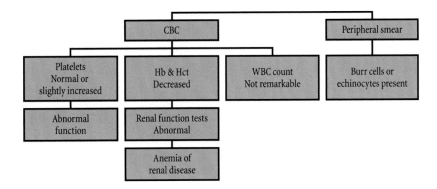

ENDOCRINE DISEASES

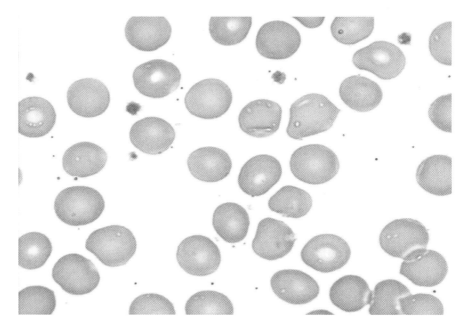

Figure **IIA8-2**

Peripheral blood smear.

Clinical Features

- ■ Symptoms are specific to the type of endocrine disorder
  - ■ Hyperthyroidism
  - ■ Hypothyroidism
  - ■ Hypercortisolism
  - ■ Hypocortisolism
  - ■ Hypoandrogenemia
  - ■ Diabetes mellitus

Pathology

- Hyperthyroidism
  - Elevated red blood cell mass secondary to enhanced BFU-E proliferation
  - Increased requirement for folic acid to accommodate the increased red blood cell production
- Hypothyroidism
  - Reduced red blood cell mass secondary to decreased oxygen requirements
- Hypercortisolism
  - Modest polycythemic state due to increased androgens
- Hypocortisolism
  - Hemoconcentrated state with a normal to slightly increased hematocrit level due to lack of the salt-retaining hormones
- Hypogonadism
  - Anemia due to reduced level of androgens
- Diabetes mellitus
  - Acute hemolysis may occur in ketoacidosis

Laboratory Features

- Hyperthyroidism
  - Macrocytic anemia
- Hypothyroidism
  - Usually macrocytic anemia
  - Iron-deficient anemia may occur when menorrhagia is present
- Hypercortisolism
  - Modest polycythemic picture
- Hypocortisolism
  - Normal or slightly increased hematocrit level
- Hyperandrogenemia
  - Slight normocytic/normochromic anemia
- Diabetes mellitus
  - Falsely elevated hematocrit level

Diagnostic Scheme

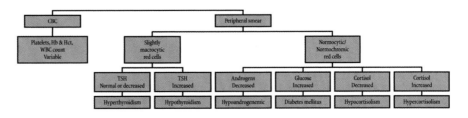

LIVER DISEASE

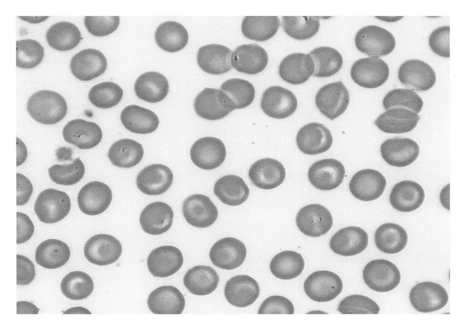

Figure IIA8-3   Peripheral blood smear.

Clinical Features

- Anemia is secondary to the abnormalities in liver function
- The most common cause of nonmegaloblastic, macrocytic anemia
- Occurs in about 50% of patients with liver disease

Pathology

- Multifaceted
  - Hemolysis
  - Impaired bone marrow response
  - Folate deficiency
  - Blood loss
- Abnormalities in red blood cell membrane lipid composition are common

Laboratory Features

White Blood Cells

■ Neutropenia, neutrophilia, or lymphopenia

Platelets

■ Decreased
■ Abnormal function

Red Blood Cells

■ Mild to moderate anemia
  ■ Macrocytic
  ■ Normocytic
  ■ Microcytic
■ Round macrocytes
■ Target cells, spur cells, acanthocytes
■ Increased reticulocytes

Bone Marrow

■ Normocellular or hypercellular with erythroid hyperplasia
■ Vacuolization of red blood cell precursors

Diagnostic Scheme

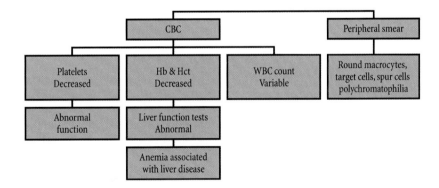

SYSTEMIC LUPUS ERYTHEMATOSUS

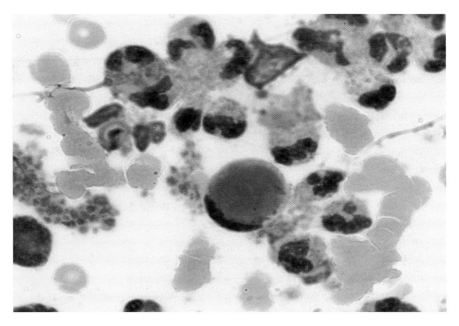

Figure IIA8-4   Buffy coat smear.

Clinical Features

- Low-grade fever
- Arthritis and arthralgia
- Skin lesions
- Nervous system disorders (psychological and neurologic changes)
- Pericarditis
- Pleuritic chest pain
- Anorexia, nausea, vomiting, and abdominal pain
- Hepatomegaly

Pathology

- Decreased cellular immunity
- Circulating immune complexes may cause tissue injury in many organ systems

Laboratory Features

White Blood Cells

■ Decreased count but usually $>2.0 \times 10^9/L$

Differential

■ Normal

Platelets

■ Decreased

Red Blood Cells

■ Normocytic/normochromic anemia
■ Hemolysis
  ■ Autoantibodies
■ Circulating anticoagulants may cause prolongation of partial thromboplastin times
■ Antinuclear antibodies may be present and may result in the presence of lupus erythematosus cells
■ Complement levels decreased

Diagnostic Scheme

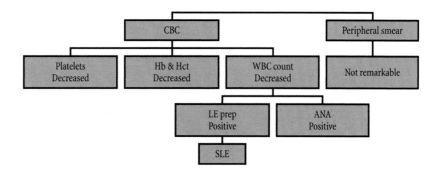

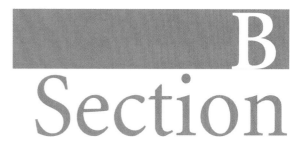

Section

White Blood Cell Disorders

CHAPTER

1

Nonmalignant Leukocyte Disorders

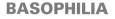

BASOPHILIA

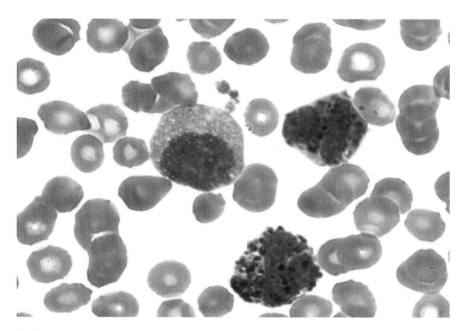

Figure **IIB1-1**   Peripheral blood smear.

Clinical Features

- Defined as >0.15 × 10^9/L basophils
- Varies with the etiology
    - Hypothyroidism with myxedema
    - Myeloproliferative disorders
        - Chronic myelogenous leukemia
        - Polycythemia vera
        - Chronic idiopathic myelofibrosis
    - After radiation exposure

Pathology

- Associated with immediate hypersensitivity reactions
    - When IgE binds to the basophil receptors, the cell degranulates and releases histamine and other inflammatory mediators
- Specific to the disorders that cause the secondary basophilia

Laboratory Features

White Blood Cells

■ Increased numbers of basophils

Red Blood Cells

■ Variable

Platelets

■ Variable

Diagnostic Scheme

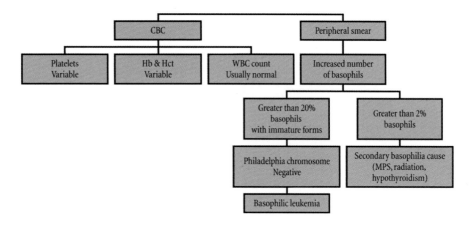

CHÉDIAK-HIGASHI ANOMALY

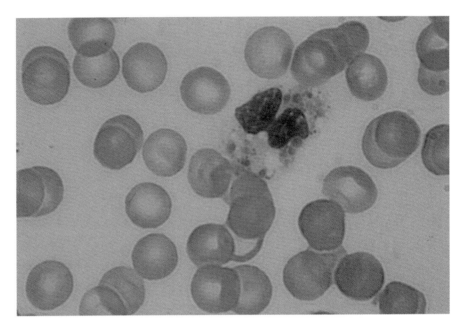

Figure **IIB1-2**   Peripheral blood smear.

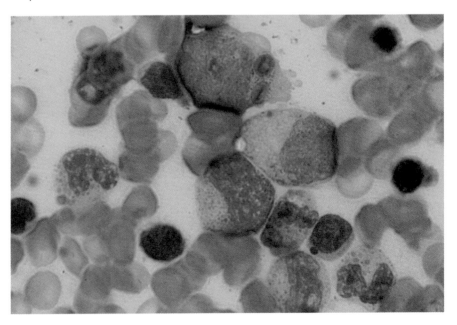

Figure **IIB1-3**   Bone marrow smear.

Clinical Features

- Increased susceptibility to bacterial infections
- Fever
- Silvery-white hair
- Photophobia
- Enlarged lymph nodes
- Hepatosplenomegaly

Pathology

- Autosomal recessive inherited disorder of granule production
- Produces serious abnormalities in the function of affected phagocytes
  - Bacterial killing is impaired
  - Degranulation is delayed and incomplete
  - Chemotaxis is defective
- Lymphocytes show an impairment of both antibody-dependent and natural killer cell–mediated cytotoxicity

Laboratory Features

White Blood Cells

- Typical count of $1-3 \times 10^9$/L
- Giant gray-green peroxidase-positive bodies are found in the cytoplasm of leukocytes
- Neutropenia

Red Blood Cells

- Normal

Platelets

- Thrombocytopenia
- Aggregation is abnormal

Coagulation studies

- Bleeding time is abnormal

Bone Marrow

- The abnormal granules from precursor vacuoles undergo fusion

Diagnostic Scheme

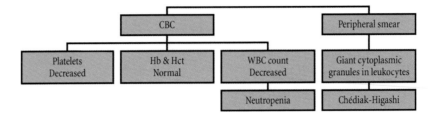

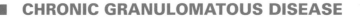

CHRONIC GRANULOMATOUS DISEASE

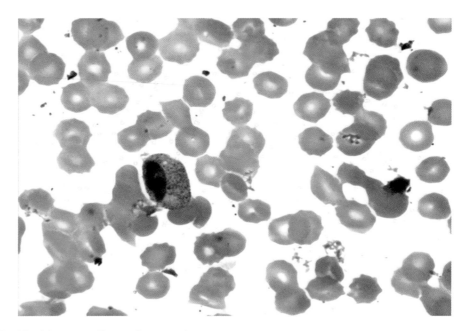

Figure IIB1-4

Nitroblue tetrazolium stain—negative.

Clinical Features

- Recurrent bacterial and fungal infections during the first 12 months of life
- Lymphadenitis
- Deep tissue infections
- Infected eczemalike rash
- Visceral and hepatic abscesses
- Recurrent pulmonary infections
- Organomegaly

Pathology

- May be inherited as an X-linked or as an autosomal recessive trait
- Failure in the activation of the respiratory burst
- Formation of granulomas during chronic inflammatory reactions

Laboratory Features

White Blood Cells

- Neutrophilia
- Nitroblue tetrazolium reduction test results negative
    - In this test, neutrophils are incubated in the presence of nitroblue tetrazolium along with an activating agent
    - The superoxide that is released reduces the dye to an insoluble dark blue formazan that can be seen as a granular precipitate in the neutrophils (see positive control)

Red Blood Cells

- Not remarkable

Platelets

- Not remarkable

Diagnostic Scheme

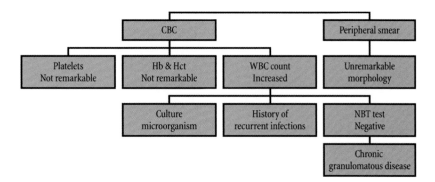

EOSINOPHILIA

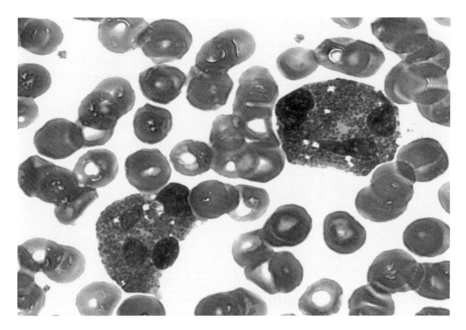

Figure **IIB1-5**   Peripheral blood smear.

Clinical Features

■ Depends on the etiology—may see fever, skin rash, adenopathy, cough, pulmonary infiltrates, muscle pain, hepatosplenomegaly

Pathology

■ Absolute eosinophil count of $>0.6 \times 10^9$/L
■ Causes include:
  ■ Parasitic infection
  ■ Allergic reaction
  ■ Respiratory disorders
  ■ Neoplastic diseases
  ■ Inflammatory or autoimmune diseases
  ■ Skin disorders

Laboratory Features

White Blood Cells

- Count normal to increased
- Eosinophils increased

Red Blood Cells

- Not remarkable

Platelets

- Not remarkable

Diagnostic Scheme

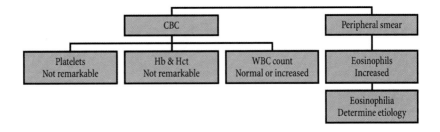

INFECTIOUS MONONUCLEOSIS

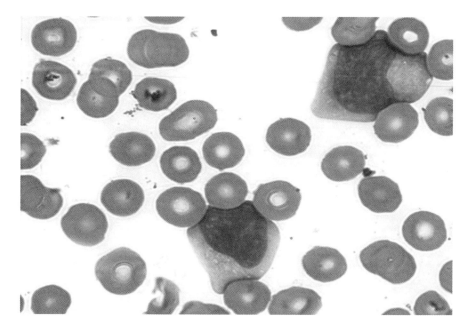

Figure IIB1-6   Peripheral blood smear.

Clinical Features

- Usually occurs in young adults aged 14–24 years
- Lethargy, anorexia, nausea, headache, chills, fever, pharyngitis, lymphadenopathy, splenomegaly, hepatomegaly
- Usually self-limited

Pathology

- Epstein-Barr virus attaches to the B lymphocytes by means of a specific Epstein-Barr virus receptor on the lymphocyte membrane
- B lymphocytes and lymphoid tissues throughout the body are involved
- Incubation period is about 30–50 days

Laboratory Features

White Blood Cells

- Agranulocytosis
- Proliferation of lymphocytes ($12–25 \times 10^9/L$)
- >20% reactive lymphocytes
- Immunoblasts may be present
- Plasmacytoid lymphocytes may be present

Red Blood Cells

- May have an autoimmune hemolytic anemia

Platelets

- Normal to decreased

Serologic Tests

- Paul-Bunnell heterophile antibodies positive

Diagnostic Scheme

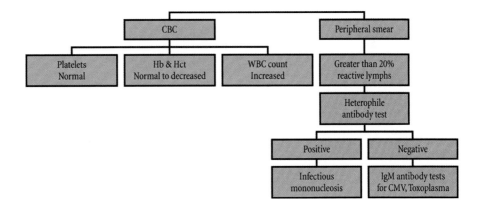

LYMPHOCYTOSIS

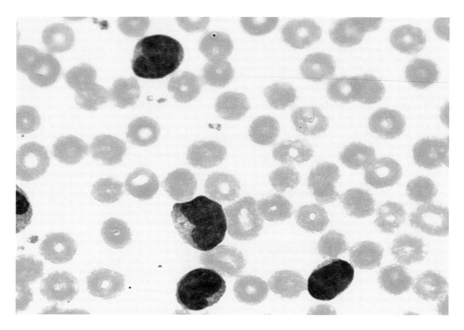

Peripheral blood smear—whooping cough.

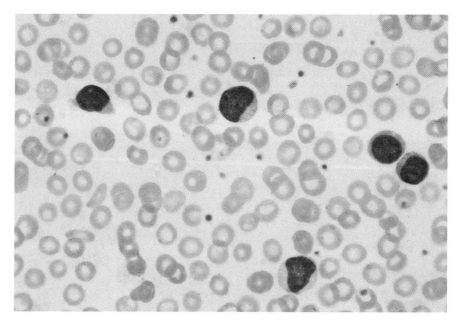

Peripheral blood smear—infectious lymphocytosis.

Clinical Features

- Absolute lymphocytosis
  - In adults, $>4.0 \times 10^9$/L
  - In children, $>7.0 \times 10^9$/L
  - In infants, $>9.0 \times 10^9$/L
- Relative lymphocytosis
  - In adults, $>45\%$
  - In children, $>70\%$
- May not be accompanied by leukocytosis
- Benign conditions
  - Viral infections
  - Bacterial infections
  - Protozoal infections
  - Other
- Malignant conditions

Bacterial Infections

- Incubation period is about 2 weeks
- Head cold, paroxysmal cough, pain in the neck and chest

Protozoal Infections (Toxoplasmosis)

- Congenital—hepatosplenomegaly, jaundice, microcephaly, mental retardation
- Acquired—lethargy, anorexia, nausea, headache, chills and fever, pharyngitis, lymphadenopathy to asymptomatic

Viral Infections (Cytomegalovirus)

- Congenital—only 10% of infected newborns show the clinical features, which include microcephaly, hepatosplenomegaly, and jaundice
- Acquired—lethargy, anorexia, nausea, headache, chills, fever, lymphadenopathy, splenomegaly, hepatomegaly

Infectious Lymphocytosis

- Usually affects young children aged 1–10 years
- Occurs in epidemics
- Incubation time is about 2–3 weeks
- Usually asymptomatic

Pathology

Bacterial Infections

- *Bordetella pertussis* infection (whooping cough)
- Usually in nonimmunized children

Protozoal Infections

- Usually the result of infection by *Toxoplasma gondii*
- Multiply in all body cells except red blood cells
- Congenital—results from placental transmission from parasitized mother
- Acquired—ingestion of oocyts from undercooked meat or inhalation from cat feces

Viral Infections

- Commonly from the cytomegalovirus
- Virus infects leukocytes, which transport it to other locations
- Virus suppresses cell-mediated immune function
- Congenital—transplacental transmission from an infected mother
- Acquired—may be spread by close contact or by blood transfusion

Infectious Lymphocytosis

- Caused by a virus, probably of the Coxsackie group
- Usually affects children younger than 10 years
- Usually no symptoms

Laboratory Features

Bacterial Infections

White Blood Cells

- Increased lymphocyte count (up to 15–56×10^9/L)

Red Blood Cells

- Not remarkable

Platelets

- Not remarkable

Protozoal Infections

White Blood Cells

- Increased
- Lymphocytosis with the presence of reactive lymphocytes
- Eosinophilia may be present

Red Blood Cells

- Hemolytic anemia

Platelets

- Variable

Serologic Tests

- Heterophile antibody test result negative

Viral Infections

White Blood Cells

- Increased
- Lymphocytosis with the presence of reactive lymphocytes

Red Blood Cells

- Hemolytic anemia

Platelets

- Variable

Serologic Tests

- Heterophile antibody test result negative

Infectious Lymphocytosis

White Blood Cells

- Usually $20.0–30.0 \times 10^9$/L
- 50–95% normal-appearing, small lymphocytes

Red Blood Cells

- Not remarkable

Platelets

- Not remarkable

Diagnostic Scheme

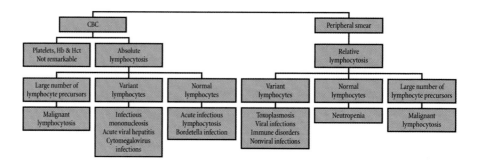

MAY-HEGGLIN ANOMALY

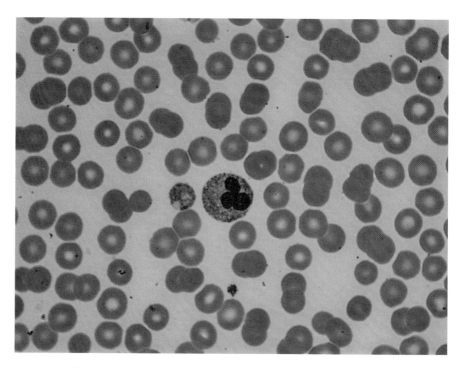

Peripheral blood smear.

Clinical Features

■ Usually a mild bleeding disorder—epistaxis, bruising, gingival bleeding, dysmenorrhea, and abnormal bleeding after dental extractions or surgery

Pathology

■ Inherited as an autosomal dominant trait affecting white blood cells and platelets

Laboratory Features

White Blood Cells

- Most neutrophils contain small homogeneous blue inclusions
- Inclusions are larger than Döhle bodies, spindle or crescent shaped, and light blue
- Found in neutrophils, eosinophils, basophils, monocytes, and occasionally even lymphocytes

Red Blood Cells

- Normal

Platelets

- Giant platelets
- Mean platelet volume increased
- Number decreased

Coagulation Studies

- Bleeding time is prolonged

Bone Marrow

- Number of megakaryocytes is normal but show some large hypergranular platelets in the cytoplasm

Diagnostic Scheme

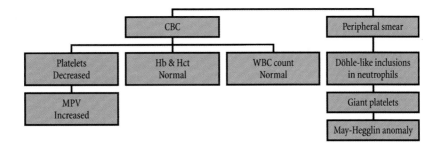

MONOCYTOSIS

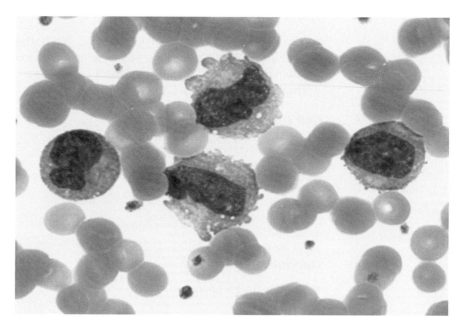

Figure IIB1-10   Peripheral blood smear.

Clinical Features

- In adults, defined as $>0.95 \times 10^9$/L monocytes
- In infants and children, defined as up to 1.0×10^9/L monocytes
- Causes of neutrophilia may be accompanied by absolute monocytosis
- Relative monocytosis may indicate a recovery from agranulocytosis or marrow hypoplasia

Pathology

- Monocytes play a role in inflammation and immune reactions
- Monocytosis is associated with several conditions
  - Tuberculosis
  - Malignancies
  - Myelodysplastic syndromes
  - Myeloproliferative syndromes
  - Lymphocytic tumors
  - Inflammatory disorders

Laboratory Features

White Blood Cells

- Increased monocytes

Red Blood Cells

- Not remarkable

Platelets

- Not remarkable

Diagnostic Scheme

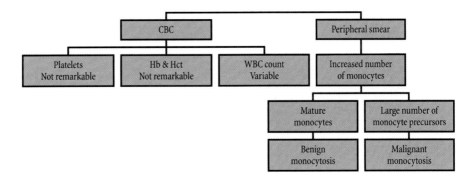

NEUTROPENIA

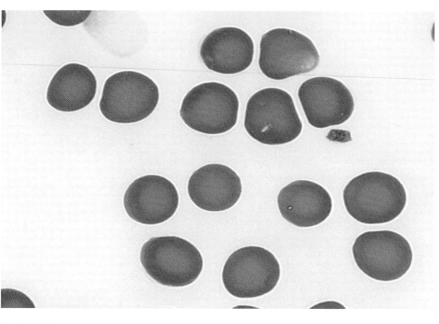

Figure **IIB1-11**   Peripheral blood smear.

Clinical Features

- Defined as an absolute neutrophil count of $<1.5 \times 10^9/L$
- May have no symptoms or may present with sudden overwhelming sepsis
  - Fever
  - Enlarged lymph nodes
  - Sternal tenderness
  - Oral lesions
- Hepatosplenomegaly

Pathology

- Decreased or ineffective production
- Reduced survival
- Abnormal distribution and sequestration

Laboratory Features

White Blood Cells

- Total number decreased
- Neutrophil count decreased

Red Blood Cells

- Not remarkable

Platelets

- Not remarkable

Diagnostic Scheme

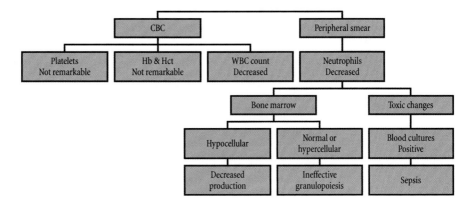

NEUTROPHILIA

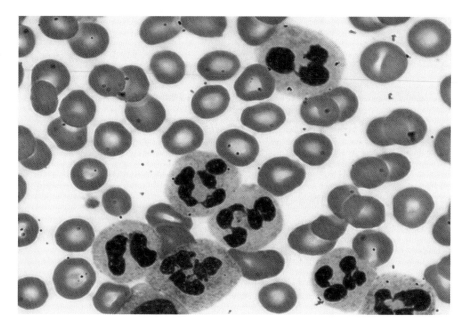

Figure IIB1-12   Peripheral blood smear.

Clinical Features

- Defined as an absolute count of $>7.0 \times 10^9/L$
- Acute neutrophilia may be caused by exercise, stress, drugs, and hormones, and the most frequent cause is bacterial infection
- Chronic neutrophilia may be seen with infection, chronic inflammation, tumors, or hematologic disorders

Pathology

- Increased production by the bone marrow
- Increased release from the marrow reserve or impaired egress from the peripheral blood
- Decreased neutrophil count in the marginating pool, with increased neutrophil count in the circulating pool
- Extreme neutrophilic reactions to severe infections or necrotizing tissue may produce a leukemoid reaction (usually $>50.0 \times 10^9/L$)
- Neoplastic disorders

Laboratory Features

White Blood Cells

- Physiologic neutrophilia
  - Increased count
- Pathologic neutrophilia
  - Increased count
  - Shift to the left
  - Vacuolization and toxic granulation
  - Döhle bodies

Red Blood Cells

- Not remarkable

Platelets

- Not remarkable

Diagnostic Scheme

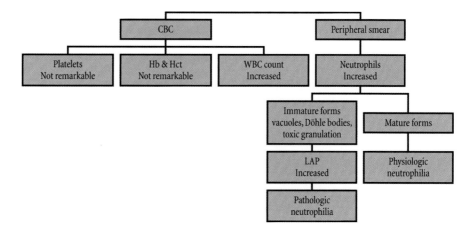

PELGER-HUËT ANOMALY

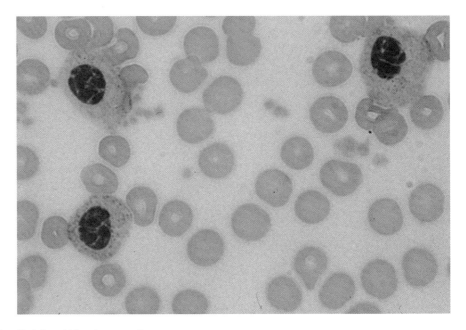

Figure IIB1-13　　Peripheral blood smear—homozygous.

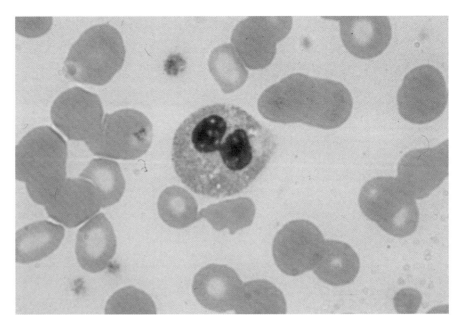

Figure IIB1-14　　Peripheral blood smear—heterozygous.

Clinical Features

- No clinical significance is associated with this anomaly

Pathology

- Inherited as an autosomal dominant trait
- Decreased segmentation of the nucleus of granulocytes
- Marked condensation of nuclear chromatin
- Normal cytoplasmic maturation

Laboratory Features

White Blood Cells

- In the heterozygous state, the granulocyte nucleus is bilobed or dumbbell shaped (Pince-Nez)
- In the homozygous state, the nucleus is round or oval (Stodtmeister)

Red Blood Cells

- Not remarkable

Platelets

- Not remarkable

Diagnostic Scheme

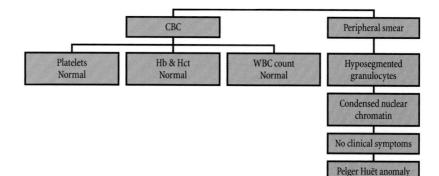

CHAPTER

2

Leukemias

ACUTE BASOPHILIC LEUKEMIA

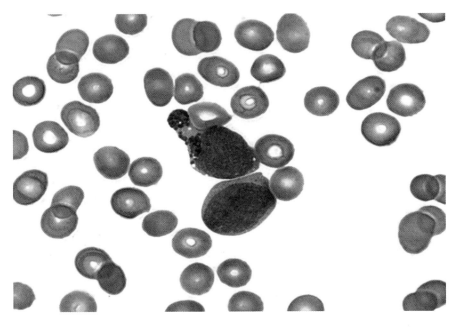

Figure **IIB2-1**   Peripheral blood smear.

Clinical Features

- Occurs in middle age
- Slight male predominance
- Weakness, fatigue, fever, wheezing, urticaria , diarrhea, pruritus, hepatosplenomegaly

Pathology

- May be a variant of chronic myelogenous leukemia
- Extremely rare condition—<1% of all acute myelogenous leukemias
- Release of basophil granules may cause shock or severe disseminated intravascular coagulation
- No consistent chromosome abnormalities

Laboratory Features

White Blood Cells

- Normal to increased
- Increased basophils
- Abnormal basophils that resemble mast cells

Red Blood Cells

- Normocytic/normochromic anemia

Platelets

- Decreased

Bone Marrow

- Increased basophils
  - 40–80% with some immature forms

Cytochemistry

- Myeloperoxidase and Sudan black B positive
- Toluidine blue positive

Immunophenotype

- Myeloid markers present (CD9, C13, CD33)
- May be positive for CD34 and class II HLA-DR

Diagnostic Scheme

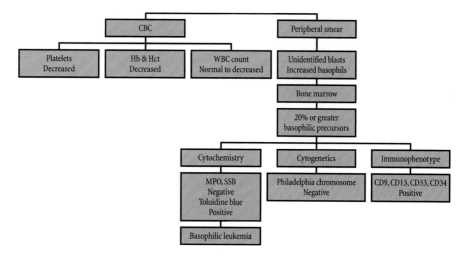

ACUTE LEUKEMIA OF AMBIGUOUS LINEAGE (BIPHENOTYPIC LEUKEMIA)

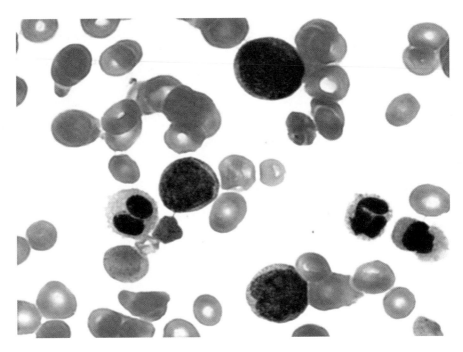

Figure IIB2-2   Peripheral blood smear.

Clinical Features

- Accounts for about 4% of acute leukemias
- More frequent in adults
- Associated with fatigue, infections, and bleeding disorders

Pathology

- Exact etiology is unknown but may be associated with toxins and radiation exposure
- Possible genetic misprogramming
- Leukemic clone could represent a bipotential cell

Laboratory Features

White Blood Cells

■ Blasts coexpress myeloid and T- or B-cell–specific antigens

Red Blood Cells

■ Normocytic/normochromic anemia

Platelets

■ Decreased

Immunophenotype

■ CD13, CD14, CD15, and/or CD33 positive with myeloid line
■ CD19, CD10, CD7, and/or CD2 positive with lymphoid line

Diagnostic Scheme

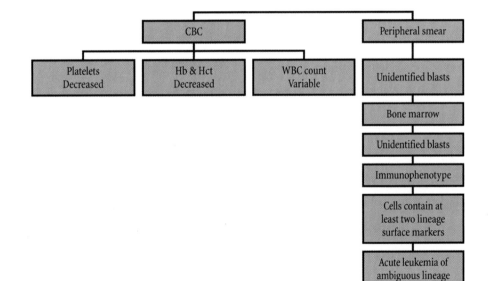

ACUTE MEGAKARYOBLASTIC LEUKEMIA (M7)

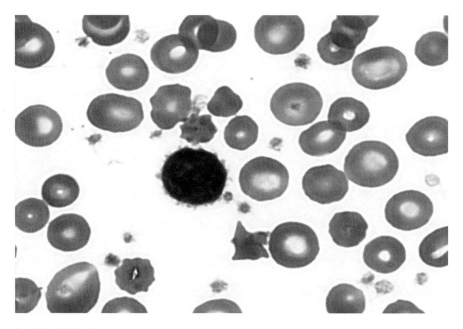

Figure **IIB2-3**   Peripheral blood smear.

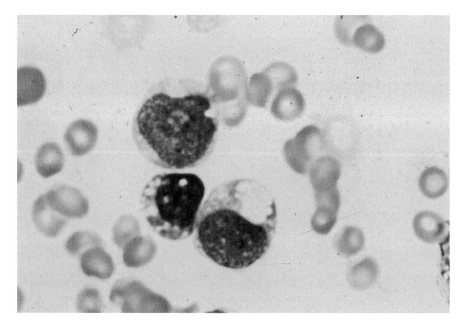

Figure **IIB2-4**   Bone marrow smear.

Clinical Features

- Pallor, fatigue, and weakness from anemia
- Bleeding, bruising, and petechial hemorrhages caused by thrombocytopenia
- Infections that fail to respond to appropriate therapy
- Bone tenderness, hepatosplenomegaly, and lymphadenopathy

Pathology

- 3–5% of myeloid leukemias
- No specific chromosome abnormalities but t(1;22) has been observed in some

Laboratory Features

White Blood Cells

- Variable but usually decreased

Red Blood Cells

- Normocytic/normochromic anemia
- Dacryocytes

Platelets

- Variable
- Bizarre and atypical

Bone Marrow

- Megakaryoblasts are highly pleomorphic
- Increased reticulum fibrosis (often a dry tap)
- Increased megakaryocytes
- ≥20% blasts
- ≥50% megakaryocytic cells

Cytochemistry

- Myeloperoxidase and Sudan black B negative
- Periodic acid–Schiff positive
- Nonspecific esterase (acetate) positive
- Nonspecific esterase (butyrate) negative

Electron Microscopy

- Platelet peroxidase positive

Immunophenotype

- CD41 and/or CD61 positive
- CD42 may be positive if the cell is more mature
- Platelet GPIIIa and von Willebrand factor positive
- CD34 and CD45 often negative

Diagnostic Scheme

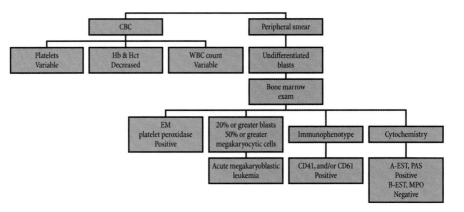

ACUTE MYELOGENOUS LEUKEMIA MINIMALLY DIFFERENTIATED (M0)

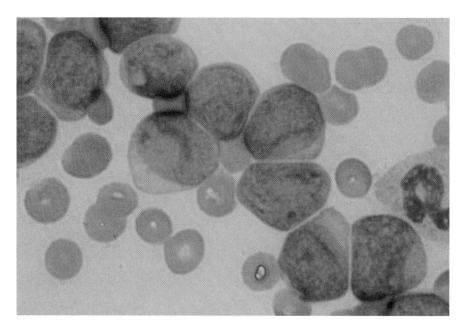

Figure IIB2-5   Bone marrow smear.

Clinical Features

- Pallor, fatigue, and weakness from anemia
- Bleeding, bruising, and petechial hemorrhages caused by thrombocytopenia
- Infections that fail to respond to appropriate therapy
- Bone tenderness, hepatosplenomegaly, and lymphadenopathy

Pathology

- Chromosomal abnormalities have been associated with M0
  - 5q-, 7q-, +8, +13, and monosomy 7
- 2–3% of myeloid leukemias

Laboratory Features

White Blood Cells

- Blasts are agranular
- Blasts may resemble L2 cells

Red Blood Cells

■ Normocytic/normochromic anemia

Platelets

■ Decreased

Bone Marrow

■ ≥20% myeloblasts—majority Type I
■ No Auer rods

Cytochemistry

■ <3% of blasts are positive with myeloperoxidase, Sudan black B, and specific esterase (chloroacetate)

Immunophenotype

■ ≥20% blasts react with any myeloid antigens (CD33, CD34, CD117, and HLA-DR)
■ Required immunophenotyping to exclude lymphoid lineage
    ■ Negative for lymphoid antigens (CD3, CD5, CD10, CD19, CD20, CD22)

Diagnostic Scheme

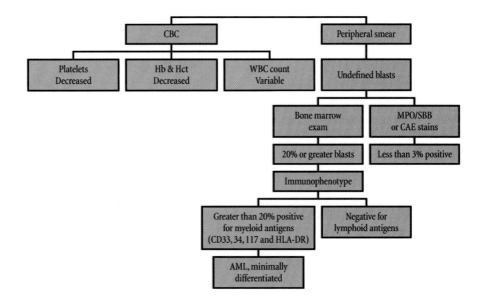

ACUTE MYELOGENOUS LEUKEMIA WITH ABNORMAL BONE MARROW EOSINOPHILS (M4Eo)

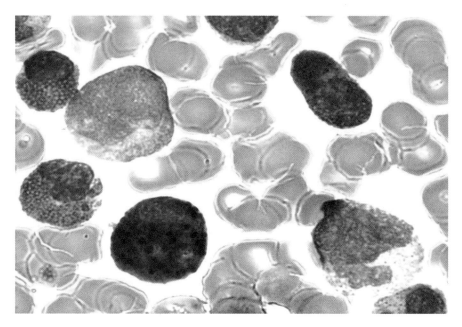

Figure IIB2-6   Bone marrow smear.

Clinical Features

- Also known as M4 with eosinophilia (FAB)
- Pallor, fatigue, and weakness from anemia
- Bleeding, bruising, and petechial hemorrhages caused by thrombocytopenia
- Infections that fail to respond to appropriate therapy
- Bone tenderness, hepatosplenomegaly, and lymphadenopathy

Pathology

- About 10–12% of the myeloid leukemias
- inv (16)
- Occurs in all age groups but predominates in younger patients
- Combination of acute myelomonocytic leukemia with abnormal eosinophils in bone marrow

Laboratory Features

White Blood Cells

■ Increased
■ Abnormal eosinophils not usually found on peripheral smear

Red Blood Cells

■ Normocytic/normochromic anemia

Platelets

■ Decreased

Bone Marrow

■ Abnormal eosinophils with monocytic or pseudo-Pelger-Huët features account for ≥5% of the nonerythroid nucleated cells
■ Large, atypical basophilic granules and eosinophilic granules within the same cell

Cytochemistry

■ Periodic acid–Schiff and specific esterase (chloroacetate) positive in the abnormal eosinophils

Diagnostic Scheme

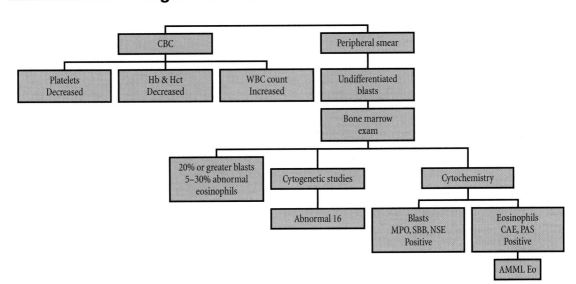

ACUTE MYELOGENOUS LEUKEMIA WITH MATURATION (M2)

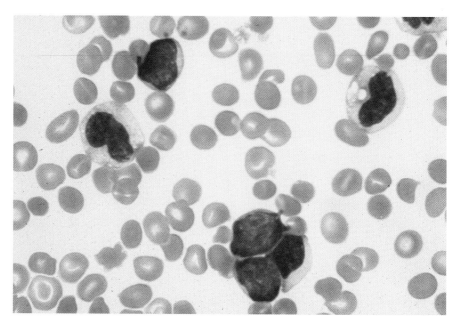

Figure **IIB2-7**   Peripheral blood smear.

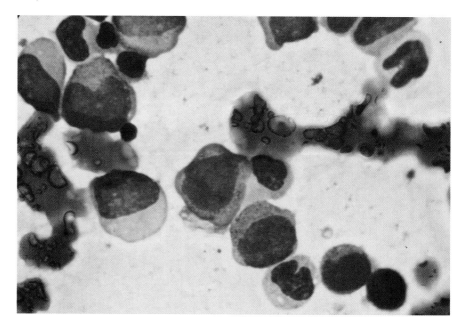

Figure **IIB2-8**   Bone marrow smear.

Clinical Features

- Pallor, fatigue, and weakness from anemia
- Bleeding, bruising, and petechial hemorrhages caused by thrombocytopenia
- Infections that fail to respond to appropriate therapy
- Bone tenderness, hepatosplenomegaly, and lymphadenopathy

Pathology

- Usually occurs in two age groups
  - <25 years
  - >60 years
- Accounts for about 30–45% of myeloid leukemias
- Chromosomal abnormalities
  - −7, −5, +4, +8, and del (5q)
  - Approximately 25% are t(8;21)
  - Categorized as acute myelogenous leukemia with recurrent genetic abnormalities (World Health Organization)
    - Large blasts with long-spindle Auer rods
    - Better prognosis

Laboratory Features

White Blood Cells

- Increased in about 50% of patients
- Type II myeloblasts found in peripheral blood and may be predominant cell
- Auer rods present
- May be associated with increased basophils or eosinophils

Red Blood Cells

- Normocytic/normochromic anemia

Platelets

- Usually decreased

Bone Marrow

- Hypocellular
- Myeloblasts, 20–89% of the nonerythroid nucleated cells
- Auer rods are common
- Maturation to promyelocytes and beyond is present in >10% of nucleated nonerythroid cells
- Trilineage dysplasia often present
  - Myelocytes and metamyelocytes may have abnormal morphologic characteristics
  - Nuclear/cytoplasmic maturation asynchrony
  - Pseudo–Pelger-Huët neutrophils
  - Hypogranulation or abnormal granulation

Cytochemistry

- Myeloperoxidase and Sudan black B positive
- Specific esterase positive

Immunophenotype

- Positive for myeloid markers (CD13, CD15, and/or CD33)
- May express markers for CD34, CD117, and HLA-DR

Diagnostic Scheme

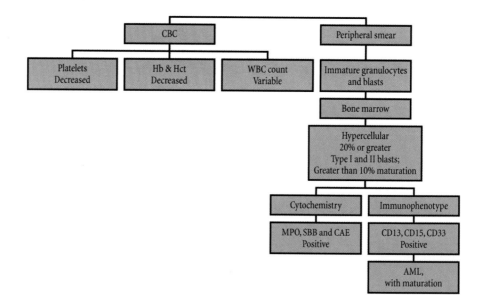

ACUTE MYELOGENOUS LEUKEMIA WITH MULTILINEAGE DYSPLASIA

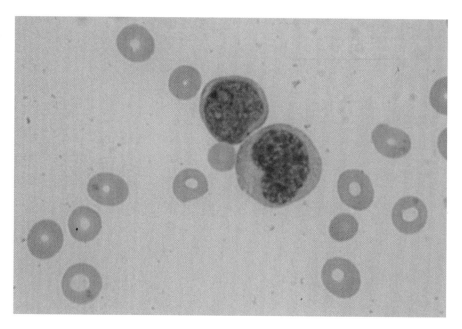

Figure **IIB2-9**   Peripheral blood smear.

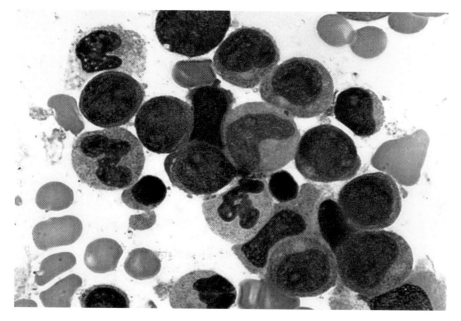

Figure **IIB2-10**   Bone marrow smear.

Clinical Features

- Usually found in the elderly
- Severe pancytopenia
- Fatigue and weakness
- Hemorrhagic symptoms
- Infection

Pathology

- Expansion of abnormal cells in the bone marrow and a decrease in normal cells
- Rearrangements of genetic material may be important in the activation of proto-oncogenes to oncogenes
- Abnormal karyotypes are seen such as -7, -5, and $+8$

Laboratory Features

White Blood Cells

- Decreased count
- Dysgranulopoiesis and dysmegakaryopoiesis

Red Blood Cells

- Anemia
- Dimorphic population
- Nucleated red blood cells

Platelets

- Decreased count

Bone Marrow

- $\geq$20% myeloblasts
- $\geq$50% dysplastic cells in two or more cell lines
- Dysgranulopoiesis
- Dysmegakaryopoiesis
- Dyserythropoiesis

Diagnostic Scheme

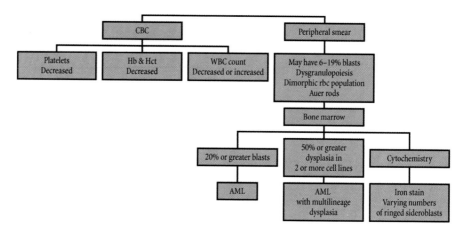

ACUTE MYELOGENOUS LEUKEMIA WITHOUT MATURATION (M1)

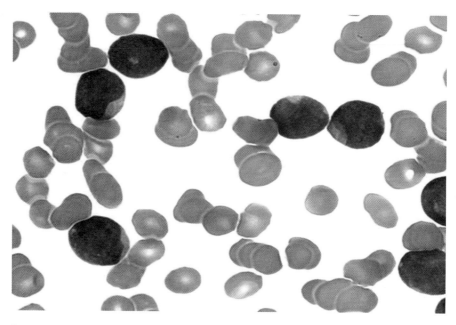

Figure IIB2-11   Peripheral blood smear.

Clinical Features

- Pallor, fatigue, and weakness from anemia
- Bleeding, bruising, and petechial hemorrhages caused by thrombocytopenia
- Infections that fail to respond to appropriate therapy
- Bone tenderness, hepatosplenomegaly, and lymphadenopathy

Pathology

- 10–20% of leukemias
- Most common in adults and infants younger than 1 year
- Chromosomal abnormalities
  - No specific associations

Laboratory Features

White Blood Cells

- Increased in 50% of patients but may be normal or decreased
- Predominant cell in peripheral blood is usually a Type I myeloblast
- Auer rods rare

Red Blood Cells

- Normocytic/normochromic anemia
- Nucleated red blood cells may be seen
- Variable anisocytosis and poikilocytosis

Platelets

- Decreased

Bone Marrow

- Hypercellular
- $\geq$20% blasts
- $\geq$90% of the nonerythroid cells are myeloblasts
- <10% promyelocytes or more mature cells and monocytes

Cytochemistry

- Myeloperoxidase and Sudan black B positive in >3% of the blasts
- Specific esterase may be positive
- Nonspecific esterases are negative

Immunophenotype

- Positive for at least two myeloid markers (CD13, CD33, and CD117)
- Negative for lymphoid markers (CD3, CD20, and CD79a)

Diagnostic Scheme

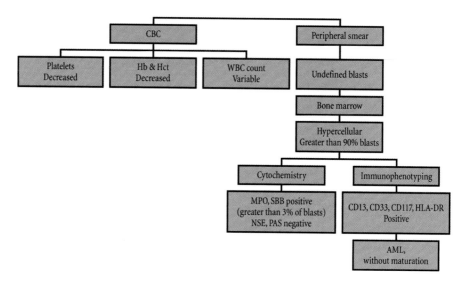

ACUTE MONOBLASTIC LEUKEMIA (M5a)

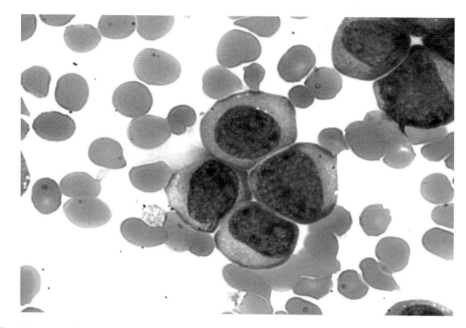

Figure IIB2-12   Peripheral blood smear.

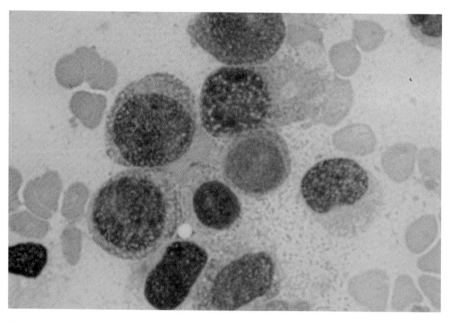

Figure IIB2-13   Bone marrow smear.

Clinical Features

- Also known as Schilling-type leukemia
- Bleeding disorder is the common presentation
- Gum hyperplasia
- Splenomegaly
- Infections
- Found in younger age groups
- Extramedullary involvement: lymph nodes, liver, skin, spleen, central nervous system

Pathology

- About 5–8% of myeloid leukemias
- Common association with abnormalities on chromosome 11 band q23

Laboratory Features

White Blood Cells

- Usually increased
- Blast morphology is variable
- Auer rods usually absent

Red Blood Cells

- Normocytic/normochromic anemia

Platelets

- Decreased

Bone Marrow

- Hypercellular
- <20% granulocytic precursors
- ≥80% are typically monoblasts
- Auer rods usually absent

Cytochemistry

- Myeloperoxidase <20% positive cells
- Nonspecific esterase ≥80% positive cells
- Nonspecific esterase with sodium fluoride inhibition ≥80% positive cells

Immunophenotype

- Variably express CD13, CD33, and CD117
- Generally show some of the markers of the monocytic line such as CD4, CD11b, CD11c, CD64, and CD36

Diagnostic Scheme

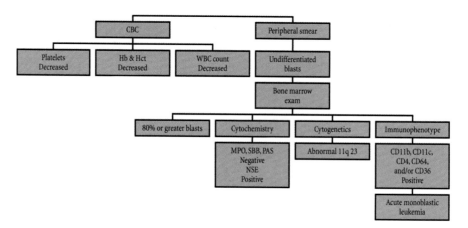

ACUTE MONOCYTIC LEUKEMIA (M5b)

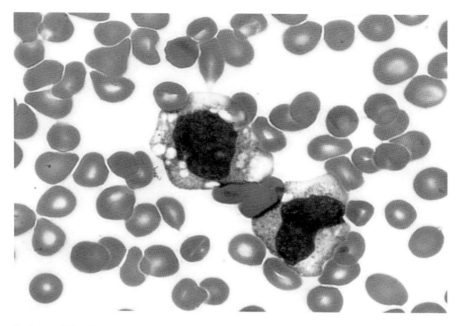

Figure IIB2-14   Peripheral blood smear.

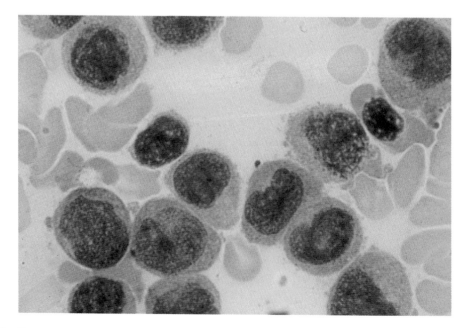

Figure IIB2-15   Bone marrow smear.

Clinical Features

- Bleeding disorder is common presentation
- Gum hyperplasia
- Splenomegaly
- Infections
- Extramedullary involvement: lymph nodes, liver, skin, spleen, central nervous system

Pathology

- Accounts for about 3–6% of myeloid leukemias
- More common in adults
- Associated with deletions and translocations involving chromosome 11 band q23

Laboratory Features

White Blood Cells

- Monocytosis
- Promonocyte is the predominant cell

Red Blood Cells

- Normocytic/normochromic anemia

Platelets

- Decreased

Bone Marrow

- ≥80% monocytic component with <80% monoblasts (usually promonocytes)
- <20% granulocytic component

Cytochemistry

- <20% myeloperoxidase positive cells
- Promonocytes may show some weak positivity with myeloperoxidase and Sudan black B negative
- ≥80% nonspecific esterase–positive cells
- ≥80% nonspecific esterase with sodium fluoride inhibition

Immunophenotype

- Variably express myeloid antigens CD13, CD33, and CD117
- May express monocytic markers CD14, CD4, CD11b, CD11c, CD36, CD64, and CD68

Diagnostic Scheme

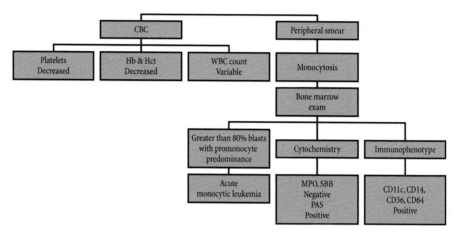

ACUTE MYELOMONOCYTIC LEUKEMIA (M4)

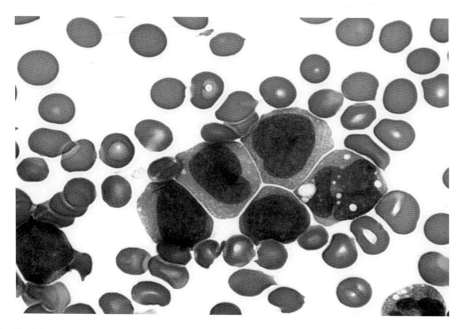

Figure IIB2-16   Peripheral blood smear.

Clinical Features

- Also known as Naegeli type
- Pallor, fatigue, and weakness from anemia
- Bleeding, bruising, and petechial hemorrhages caused by thrombocytopenia
- Infections that fail to respond to appropriate therapy
- Bone tenderness, hepatosplenomegaly, and lymphadenopathy
- Infiltration of leukemic cells in extramedullary sites
- Gingival hyperplasia is found in about 10% of cases

Pathology

- Accounts for 15–25% of acute myelogenous leukemia cases
- Usually occurs in older individuals
- Male:female ratio 1.4:1
- Nonspecific chromosome abnormalities

Laboratory Features

White Blood Cells

- Usually increased
- Both myelocytic and monocytic differentiation in peripheral blood and bone marrow
- $>5 \times 10^9$/L monocytes and precursors
- Auer rods may be present

Red Blood Cells

- Normocytic/normochromic anemia

Platelets

- Decreased but may be normal

Bone Marrow

- Resembles acute myelogenous leukemia with maturation and with blasts composing >19% and <80% of nonerythroid component
- Monocytic precursors exceed 19% and <80% of nonerythroid nucleated cells

Cytochemistry

- Myeloblasts are positive for myeloperoxidase, Sudan black B, and specific esterase and negative with nonspecific esterases
- Monoblasts are negative or only slightly positive for myeloperoxidase and negative or only finely granular with Sudan black B
- Nonspecific esterases are positive and inhibited by sodium fluoride

Immunophenotype

- Positive for the myeloid antigens—CD13 and CD33
- Positive for the monocytic markers—CD14, CD4, CD11b, CD64, and CD36

Diagnostic Scheme

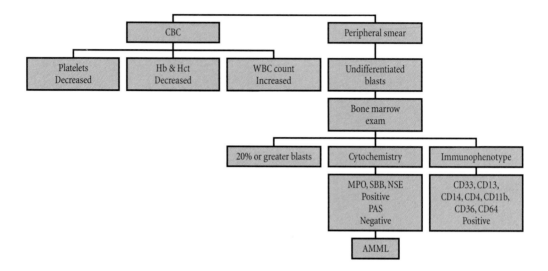

ACUTE PROMYELOCYTIC LEUKEMIA (M3)—HYPERGRANULAR

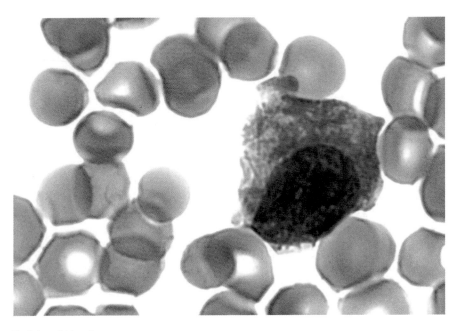

Figure **IIB2-17**   Peripheral blood smear.

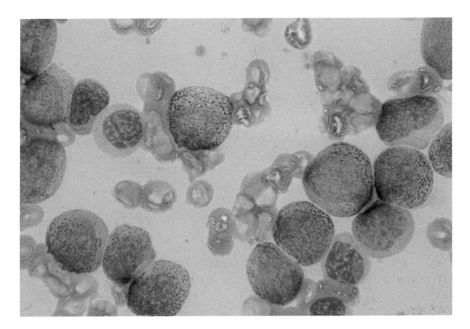

Figure **IIB2-18**   Bone marrow smear.

Clinical Features
■ Accounts for about 5–8% of acute myelogenous leukemia cases
■ Predominates in patients during mid-life
■ Common features in all types of acute myelogenous leukemias are pallor, fatigue, and weakness
■ Bleeding is the most common presenting symptom (70–80% of cases)
■ Frequently associated with disseminated intravascular coagulation
■ Two forms exist: hypergranular (70–80%) and microgranular or hypogranular (20–30%)

Pathology
■ Malignant transformation of the promyelocytes
■ Suppression of normal hematopoiesis
■ Chromosome abnormality—t (15;17)

Laboratory Features
White Blood Cells
■ Usually decreased
■ Blasts and promyelocytes show heavy granulation and multiple Auer rods

Red Blood Cells
■ Normocytic/normochromic anemia

Platelets
■ Usually decreased

Bone Marrow
■ Most of the cells are abnormal promyelocytes with heavy azurophilic granulation
■ Multiple Auer rods found in promyelocytes

Cytochemistry
■ Sudan black B, peroxidase, and specific esterase strongly positive

Immunophenotype
■ CD33 homogeneously positive
■ CD13 heterogeneously positive
■ HLA-DR and CD34 are usually negative

Diagnostic Scheme

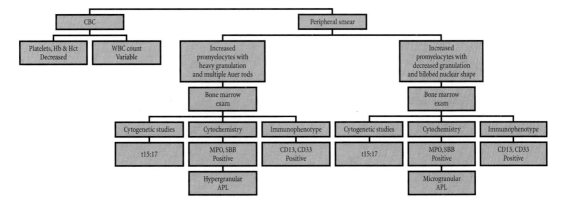

ACUTE PROMYELOCYTIC LEUKEMIA (M3)—MICROGRANULAR

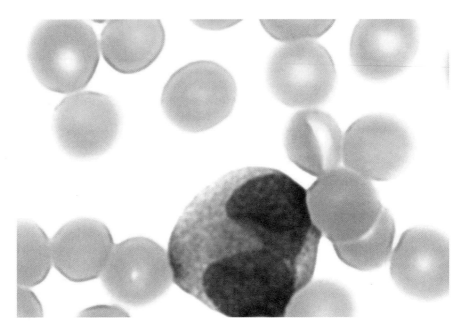

Figure **IIB2-19**   Peripheral blood smear.

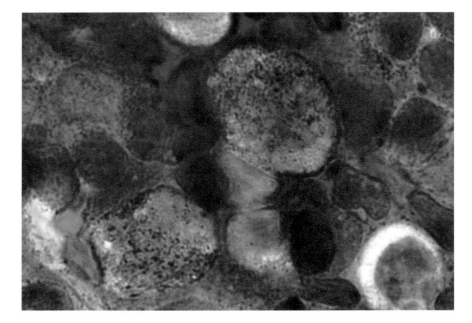

Figure **IIB2-20**   Bone marrow smear.

Clinical Features

- Accounts for about 5–8% of acute myelogenous leukemia cases
- Predominates in patients during mid-life
- Common features in all types of acute myelogenous leukemias are pallor, fatigue, and weakness
- Bleeding is the most common presenting symptom (70–80% of cases)
- Frequently associated with disseminated intravascular coagulation
- Two forms exist: hypergranular (70–80%) and microgranular or hypogranular (20–30%)

Pathology

- Malignant transformation of the promyelocytes
- Suppression of normal hematopoiesis
- Chromosome abnormality—t(15;17)

Laboratory Features

White Blood Cells

- Markedly increased
- The promyelocytes are usually bilobed and the cytoplasm contains only a few granules

Red Blood Cells

- Normocytic/normochromic anemia

Platelets

- Usually decreased

Bone Marrow

- Promyelocytes found in the microgranular type are very similar to those in the hypergranular type
- Multiple Auer rods found in promyelocytes

Cytochemistry

- Sudan black B, peroxidase, and specific esterase strongly positive

Immunophenotype

- CD33 homogeneously positive
- CD13 heterogeneously positive
- HLA-DR and CD34 are usually negative

Diagnostic Scheme

See ACUTE PROMYELOCYTIC LEUKEMIA (M3)—HYPERGRANULAR

BURKITT'S LYMPHOMA

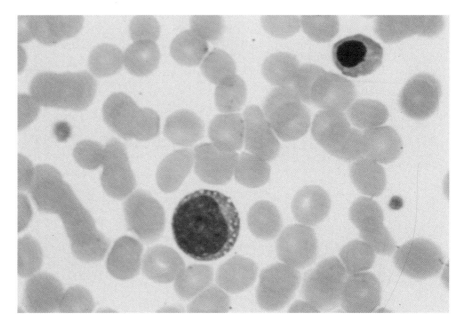

Figure IIB2-21   Peripheral blood smear.

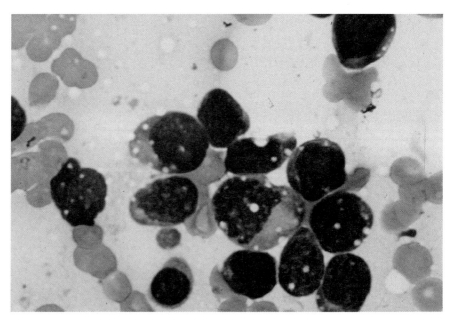

Figure IIB2-22   Bone marrow smear.

Clinical Features

- 3–4% of precursor lymphoblastic leukemias in children and adults
- May present at extranodal sites (jaw and other facial bone in about 50%)
- Involved organs are replaced by tissue where hemorrhage and necrosis have taken place; adjacent organs are compressed and/or infiltrated
- May be seen as an acute leukemia (L3)
- Three clinical variants
  - Endemic—Most common malignancy of childhood in equatorial Africa
  - Sporadic—Found in children and young adults throughout the world
  - Immunodeficiency associated—Found in association with human immunodeficiency virus infection

Pathology

- Epstein-Barr virus is important in the endemic variant
- Other factors may also play a role, including low socioeconomic status and early Epstein-Barr virus infections
- Genetic abnormalities involving the MYC gene on chromosome 8 may also play a role
- t(8;14) is the most common chromosomal abnormality; t(8;22) is also seen

Laboratory Features

White Blood Cells

- Increased, decreased, or normal

Red Blood Cells

- Normocytic/normochromic anemia

Platelets

- Thrombocytopenia often present and severe

Cytochemistry

- Sudan black B, peroxidase, specific esterase, and nonspecific esterase negative
- Periodic acid–Schiff negative
- Terminal deoxynucleotidyl transferase negative
- Oil red O positive
- HLA-DR positive

Immunophenotype

- CD19, CD20, and sIg positive

Diagnostic Scheme

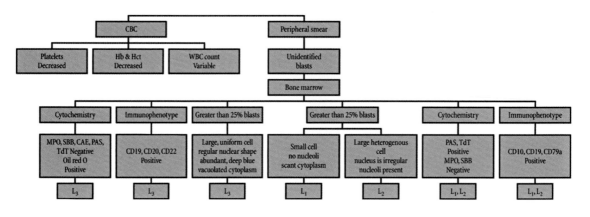

ERYTHROLEUKEMIA (M6a)

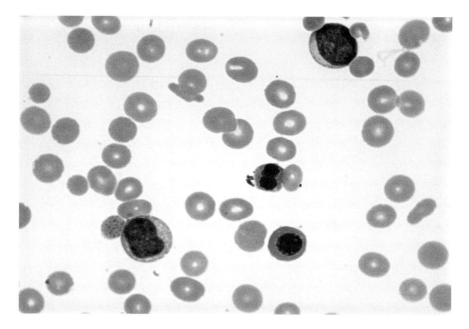

Figure **IIB2-23**   Peripheral blood smear.

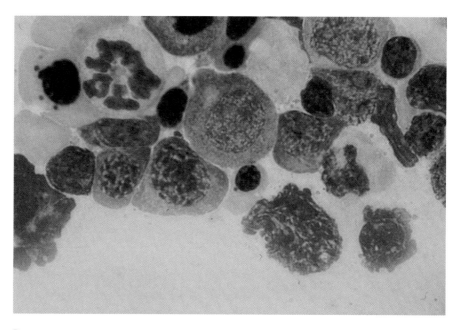

Figure **IIB2-24**   Bone marrow smear.

Clinical Features

■ Weakness, fatigue, weight loss, fever
■ Hepatosplenomegaly
■ Petechiae, purpura
■ Usually older than 50 years

Pathology

■ About 5–6% of myeloid leukemias
■ Usually exhibits three phases (more myeloid involvement as disease progresses)
   ■ Erythrymic
   ■ Mixed
   ■ Acute nonlymphocytic leukemia
■ No specific chromosome abnormalities

Laboratory Features

White Blood Cells

■ Variable

Red Blood Cells

■ Normocytic/normochromic to macrocytic/normochromic anemia
■ Anisocytosis and poikilocytosis
■ Basophilic stippling
■ Nucleated red blood cells

Platelets

■ Variable

Bone Marrow

■ ≥50% erythroblasts of all nucleated cells
■ ≥20% myeloblasts of nonerythroid cells
■ Erythroid hyperplasia
■ Megaloblastoid changes
■ Dyserythropoietic changes
■ Dysgranulopoietic changes

Cytochemistry

- Periodic acid–Schiff positive in early erythrocytic precursors
- Myeloperoxidase and Sudan black B show >5% positive in myeloblasts

Immunophenotype

- CD13, CD33, and CD117 positive in myeloid component
- Glycophorin A positive in erythroid component

Diagnostic Scheme

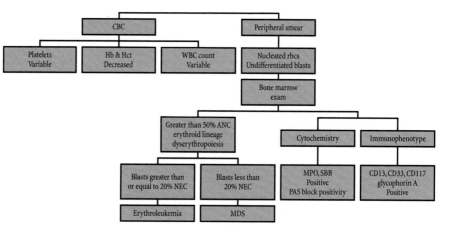

PRECURSOR LYMPHOBLASTIC LEUKEMIA (L1)

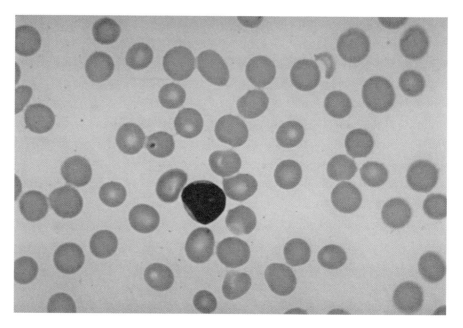

Figure **IIB2-25**   Peripheral blood smear.

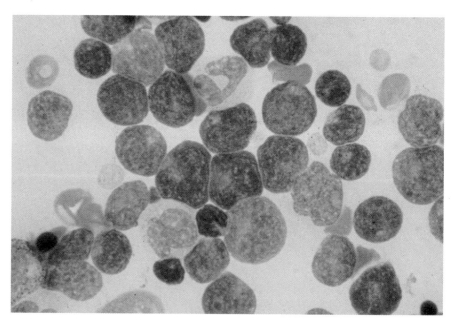

Figure **IIB2-26**   Bone marrow smear.

Clinical Features

- Onset is abrupt
- Fatigue, pallor, weight loss, and anorexia
- Petechiae or ecchymoses, bone pain
- Occasionally central nervous system symptoms (headache)
- Splenomegaly, hepatomegaly, and lymphadenopathy
- About 80% of cases are in children
  - Peak ages, 2–5 years

Pathology

- Mutation of a single lymphoid stem cell causing proliferation of malignant lymphoblasts
- Replacement of normal hematopoietic tissue in the bone marrow by the abnormal clone
- Infiltration of the lymph nodes, spleen, liver, and other organs with lymphoblasts
- Chromosome abnormalities are more common in precursor B-ALL
  - t(9;22) (q34-q11.2)
  - t(4;11) (q21;q23)
  - t(1;19) (q23;p13.3)
  - t(12;21)(p13;q22)
  - Hyperdiploid >50%
  - Hypodiploid

Laboratory Features

White Blood Cells

- Increased, decreased, or normal

Red Blood Cells

- Normocytic/normochromic anemia

Platelets

- Thrombocytopenia often present and severe

Bone Marrow

- Hypercellular
- >25% blasts
- Predominantly small blasts, up to twice the size of a normal small lymphocyte

- Nucleoli not present
- Cytoplasm is scant and only slightly or moderately basophilic

Cytochemistry

- Sudan black B, peroxidase, specific esterase, and nonspecific esterase negative
- Block positivity with periodic acid–Schiff
- Terminal deoxynucleotidyl transferase positive
- HLA-DR positive

Immunophenotype

- CD19 and CD20 positive
- CD10 positive or negative

Diagnostic Scheme

See BURKITT'S LYMPHOMA

PRECURSOR LYMPHOBLASTIC LEUKEMIA—L2

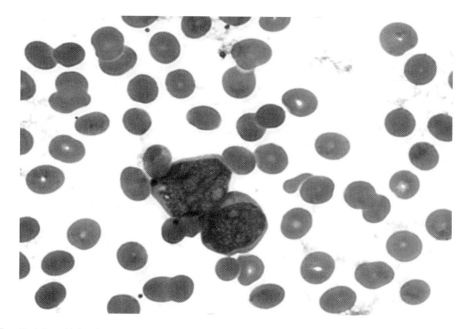

Figure **IIB2-27**   Peripheral blood smear.

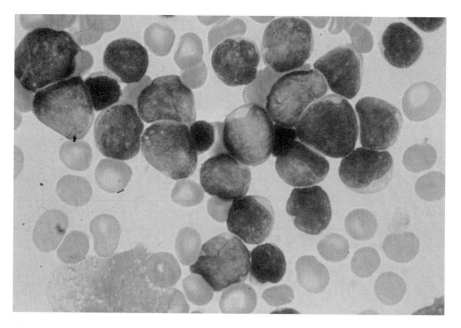

Figure **IIB2-28**   Bone marrow smear.

Clinical Features

- Onset is abrupt
- Fatigue, pallor, weight loss, and anorexia
- Petechiae or ecchymoses, bone pain
- Occasionally central nervous system symptoms (headache)
- Splenomegaly, hepatomegaly, and lymphadenopathy
- Majority of adult cases

Pathology

- Mutation of a single lymphoid stem cell causing proliferation of malignant lymphoblasts
- Replacement of normal hematopoietic tissue in the bone marrow by the abnormal clone
- Infiltration of the lymph nodes, spleen, liver, and other organs with lymphoblasts
- Chromosome abnormalities are more common in precursor B-ALL
  - t(9;22) (q34-q11.2)
  - t(4;11) (q21;q23)
  - t(1;19) (q23;p13.3)
  - t(12;21) (p13;q22)
  - Hyperdiploid >50%
  - Hypodiploid

Laboratory Features

White Blood Cells

- Increased, decreased, or normal

Red Blood Cells

- Normocytic/normochromic anemia

Platelets

- Thrombocytopenia often present and severe

Bone Marrow

- Larger blasts than in L1
- Heterogeneous in size
- Nucleus is irregular with clefting
- Nucleoli are present

Cytochemistry

■ Sudan black B, peroxidase, specific esterase, and nonspecific esterase negative
■ Block positivity with periodic acid–Schiff
■ Terminal deoxynucleotidyl transferase positive
■ HLA-DR positive

Immunophenotype

■ CD19 and CD20 positive
■ CD10 positive or negative

Diagnostic Scheme

See BURKITT'S LYMPHOMA

PURE ERYTHROID LEUKEMIA (M6b)

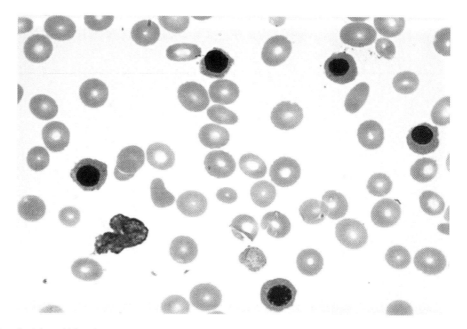

Figure **IIB2-29**   Peripheral blood smear.

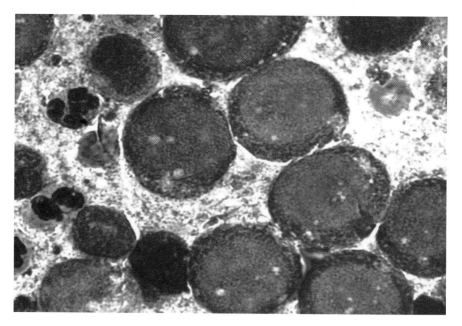

Figure **IIB2-30**   Bone marrow smear.

Clinical Features

- Weakness, fatigue, weight loss, and fever
- Hepatosplenomegaly
- Petechiae and purpura
- Extremely rare but can occur at any age

Pathology

- Erythroid cell line malignancy with no myeloid involvement
- No specific chromosome abnormalities

Laboratory Features

White Blood Cells

- Variable

Red Blood Cells

- Usually a macrocytic anemia

Platelets

- Decreased

Bone Marrow

- >80% cells are of erythroid lineage
- No evidence of myeloblastic component

Cytochemistry

- Myeloperoxidase, nonspecific esterase, and Sudan black B negative
- Block positivity with periodic acid–Schiff

Immunophenotype

- Carbonic anhydrase 1 and glycophorin A positive

Diagnostic Scheme

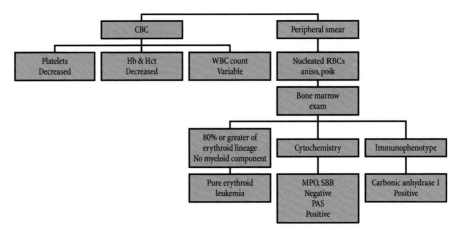

CHAPTER

3

Myelodysplastic Syndromes

MYELODYSPLASTIC SYNDROME WITH ISOLATED DEL (5q-) CHROMOSOME ABNORMALITY

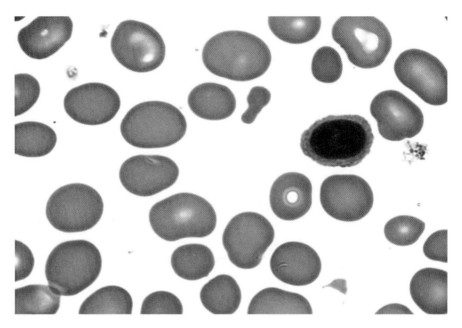

Figure IIB3-1   Peripheral blood smear.

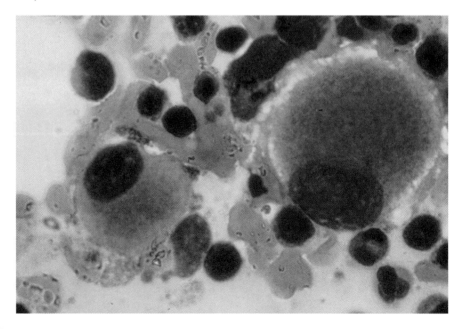

Figure IIB3-2   Bone marrow smear.

Clinical Features

- Also known as 5q-syndrome
- Usually occurs in older females
- Symptoms progress from anemia to hemorrhage and infection
- Fatigue and weakness may be the presenting symptoms

Pathology

- Loss of a portion of the long arm of chromosome 5
- Loss of genes for granulocyte-macrophage colony-stimulating factor, macrophage colony-stimulating factor, interleukin 3, and platelet-derived growth factor receptor or other growth factors may lead to this syndrome

Laboratory Features

White Blood Cells

- Count decreased
- Neutropenia
- <5% blasts

Red Blood Cells

- Macrocytic anemia
- Hemoglobin level often <8.0 g/dL

Platelets

- Normal or increased

Bone Marrow

- <5% blasts
- Hypolobulated megakaryocytes
- Hypercellular or normocellular
- May have dysplastic erythroid precursors

Cytochemistry

- Prussian blue stain
  - <15% ringed sideroblasts

Diagnostic Scheme

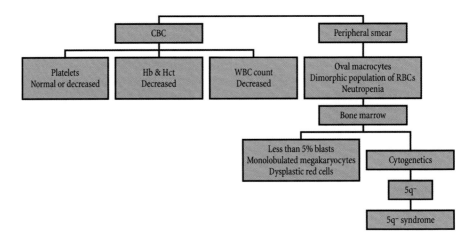

REFRACTORY ANEMIA

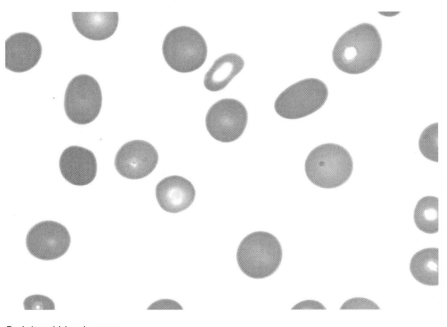

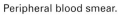

Figure **IIB3-3**   Peripheral blood smear.

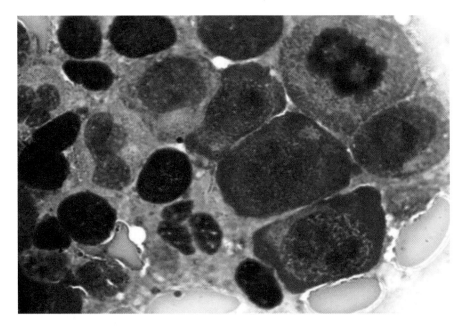

Figure **IIB3-4**   Bone marrow smear.

Clinical Features

- Usually occurs in older adults
- Pallor and fatigue
- Asymptomatic if early in the disease

Pathology

- Accounts for about 5–10% of myelodysplastic syndromes
- Abnormal group or clone of cells arise from an abnormal stem cell
- No specific acquired clonal chromosome abnormalities
    - May see del (20q), +8, abnormalities of 5, and/or 7
- Peripheral blood cytopenia is due to ineffective dyserythropoiesis

Laboratory Features

White Blood Cells

- Normal count
- <1% blasts

Red Blood Cells

- Anemia
- Oval macrocytes
- Dimorphic population
- Increased mean corpuscular volume
- Increased red blood cell distribution width

Platelets

- Normal count

Bone Marrow

- <5% blasts
- <15% ringed sideroblasts
- Cellularity normal or increased
- Erythrocytic hyperplasia with dyplasia

Chemistries

- Normal to increased iron level

Diagnostic Scheme

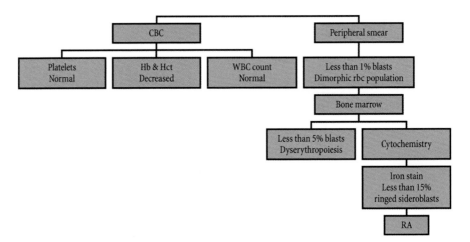

REFRACTORY ANEMIA WITH EXCESS BLASTS (RAEB-1 AND RAEB-2)

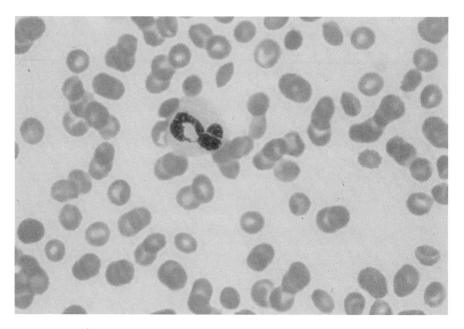

Figure **IIB3-5**   Peripheral blood smear.

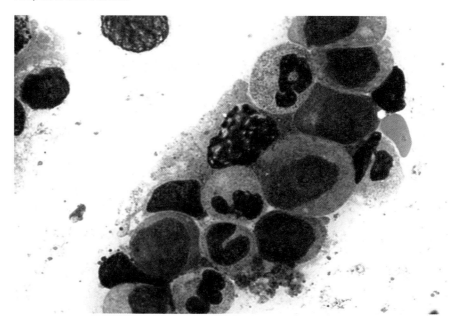

Figure **IIB3-6**   Bone marrow smear.

Clinical Features

- Occurs most commonly in older adults
- Fatigue and weakness
- Hemorrhagic symptoms
- Infection is the most common cause of death
- Hepatomegaly and splenomegaly may be present

Pathology

- Accounts for about 40% of myelodysplastic syndromes
- Expansion of abnormal cells in the bone marrow and a decrease in normal cells
- Rearrangements of genetic material may be important in the activation of proto-oncogenes to oncogenes
- May have clonal cytogenetic abnormalities
  - Most common is the deletion of the long arm of 5 (5q-)
  - Deletion of long arm of 7 (7q-)
  - Trisomy 8 (+8)

Laboratory Features

RAEB-1

White Blood Cells

- Neutropenia
- Degranulated neutrophils
- Pseudo–Pelger-Huët cells
- $<1 \times 10^9$/L monocytes
- <5% blasts

Red Blood Cells

- Anisopoikilocytosis with macrocytes
- Dimorphic population
- Decreased reticulocytes

Bone Marrow

- Hypercellular, may be hypocellular or normocellular
- Dysgranulopoiesis and/or dyserythropoiesis and/or dysmegakaryopoiesis
- May have increased number of ringed sideroblasts
- 5–9% blasts (Types I and II)
- No Auer rods

RAEB-2

White Blood Cells

- Neutropenia
- Degranulated neutrophils
- Pseudo–Pelger-Huët cells
- $<1 \times 10^9$/L monocytes

Red Blood Cells

- Anisopoikilocytosis with macrocytes
- Dimorphic population
- Decreased reticulocyte count

Platelets

- Decreased
- Large, abnormal

Bone Marrow

- Hypercellular, may be hypocellular or normocellular
- Dysgranulopoiesis and/or dyserythropoiesis and/or dysmegakaryopoiesis
- May have increased number of ringed sideroblasts
- 10–19% blasts (Type I and II)
- Auer rods may be seen

Cytochemistry

- Decreased activity of peroxidase and Sudan black B if cells are degranulated
- Prussian blue stain may show increased number of ringed sideroblasts

Diagnostic Scheme

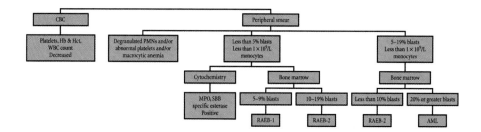

REFRACTORY ANEMIA WITH RINGED SIDEROBLASTS

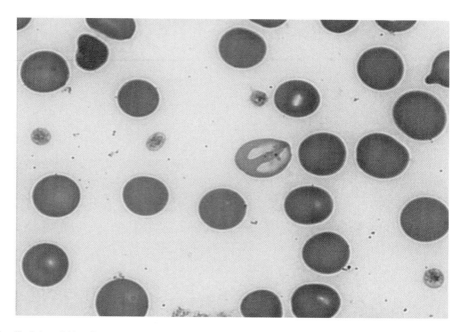

Figure IIB3-7   Peripheral blood smear.

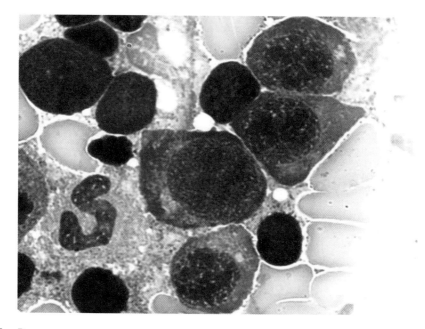

Figure IIB3-8   Bone marrow smear.

Clinical Features

- Also known as idiopathic acquired sideroblastic anemia or sideroblastic anemia
- Usually occurs in older adults
- Fatigue and pallor
- More frequent in males than females
- Liver and spleen may show evidence of iron deposition

Pathology

- Accounts for about 10–12% of myelodysplastic syndromes
- Abnormal group or clone of cells arise from an abnormal stem cell
- Peripheral blood cytopenia is secondary to ineffective cell production

Laboratory Features

White Blood Cells

- <1% blasts
- Normal count

Red Blood Cells

- Anemia
- Dimorphic picture with hypochromic microcytes and normocytic or macrocytic cells
- Occasional Pappenheimer bodies
- Decreased reticulocyte count

Platelets

- Normal count

Bone Marrow

- <5% blasts
- Dyserythropoiesis (>10% of all nucleated red blood cells)
- ≥15% ringed sideroblasts

Diagnostic Scheme

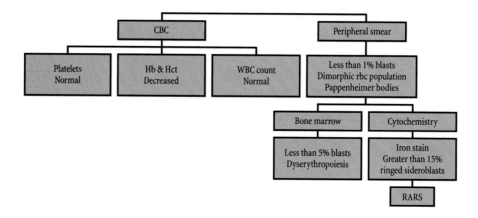

REFRACTORY CYTOPENIA WITH MULTILINEAGE DYSPLASIA

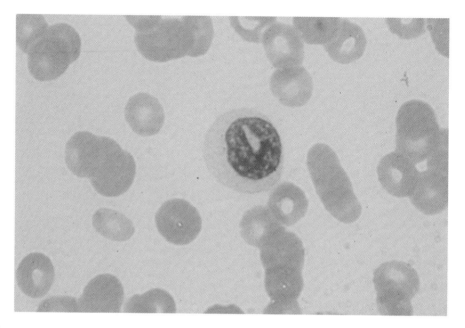

Figure **IIB3-9**   Peripheral blood smear.

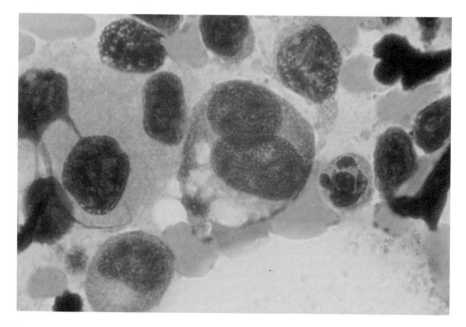

Figure **IIB3-10**   Bone marrow smear.

Clinical Features

- Occurs in older adults
- Patients present with symptoms of bone marrow failure with cytopenia in two or more myeloid lineages
    - Pallor
    - Infections
    - Bleeding

Pathology

- Accounts for about 23–25% of myelodysplastic syndromes
- Expansion of abnormal cells in the bone marrow and a decrease in normal cells
- Chromosomal abnormalities
    - Monosomy 5,7; trisomy 8; and deletions (5q), (7q), (20q)

Laboratory Features

White Blood Cells

- Hypogranulation of neutrophils
- Pseudo–Pelger-Huët nuclei
- No or rare blasts
- No Auer rods
- $<1 \times 10^9$/L monocytes

Red Blood Cells

- Decreased
- Dimorphic population

Platelets

- Normal to decreased
- May be abnormal

Bone Marrow

- Dysplasia in $\geq$10% of the cells in two or more myeloid cell lines
- $<$5% blasts
- No Auer rods

Cytochemistry

- Prussian blue stain
  - <15% ringed sideroblasts indicate refractory cytopenia with multilineage dysplasia
  - ≥15% ringed sideroblasts indicate refractory cytopenia with multilineage dysplasia with ringed sideroblasts

Diagnostic Scheme

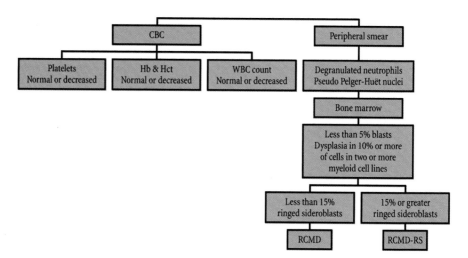

CHAPTER

4

Myeloproliferative Diseases

CHRONIC EOSINOPHILIC LEUKEMIA

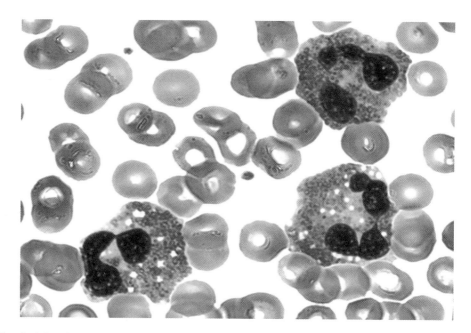

Figure IIB4-1   Peripheral blood smear.

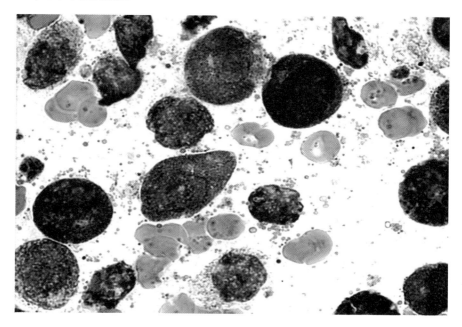

Figure IIB4-2   Bone marrow smear.

Clinical Features

- Hepatosplenomegaly
- Skin involvement
- Usually middle-aged males are affected
- Fever and weight loss
- Central nervous system irregularities, congestive heart failure, and pulmonary fibrosis

Pathology

- Rare
- Clonal abnormality
- No single chromosomal abnormalities
  - May see +8 or isochromosome 17
- Philadelphia chromosome or BCR/ABL fusion gene negative

Laboratory Features

White Blood Cells

- Persistent absolute eosinophilia ($>1.4 \times 10^9$/L)
- 30–70% eosinophils
- Count is usually $>30.0 \times 10^9$/L
- <20% blasts

Red Blood Cells

- Normocytic/normochromic anemia

Platelets

- Decreased

Bone Marrow

- Eosinophilia with increasing myeloid immaturity
- <20% blasts
- Increased number of eosinophilic myelocytes
- Increased fibrosis

Cytochemistry

■ Myeloperoxidase positive
■ Normal leukocyte alkaline phosphatase level
■ Specific esterase (chloroacetate esterase) negative

Diagnostic Scheme

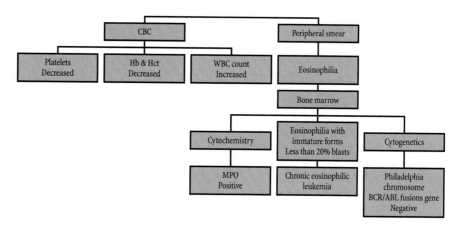

CHRONIC IDIOPATHIC MYELOFIBROSIS

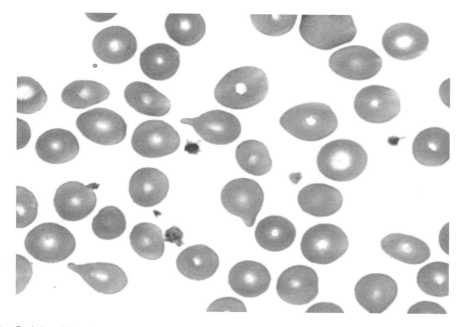

Figure IIB4-3   Peripheral blood smear.

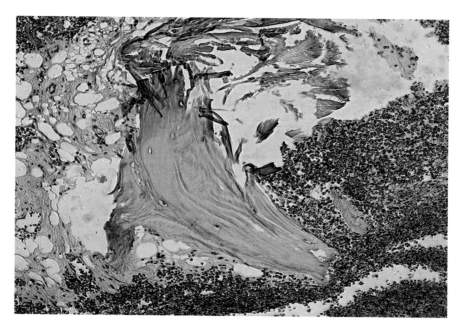

Figure IIB4-4   Bone marrow biopsy.

Clinical Features

■ Also known as agnogenic myeloid metaplasia or myelofibrosis with myeloid metaplasia
■ Occurs in elderly persons
■ Fatigue, weakness, weight loss, gouty arthritis, petechiae, and purpura
■ Lymphadenopathy
■ No or mild hepatosplenomegaly in the prefibrotic stage and moderate to marked hepatosplenomegaly in the fibrotic stage
■ Anemia and pallor

Pathology

■ Clonal stem cell disorder that involves the multipotential stem cell
■ Fibrosis is a secondary abnormality
■ Growth factors stimulate fibroblastic proliferation
■ No specific chromosomal abnormalities
  ■ May see del (13q) and (20q) and partial trisomy (1q)

Laboratory Features

General Findings

White Blood Cells

■ Count is usually $<30.0 \times 10^9/L$
■ Immature cells in the myeloid series

Red Blood Cells

■ Nucleated red blood cells
■ Normocytic/normochromic anemia
■ Dacryocytes

Platelets

■ Normal, decreased, or increased
■ Morphology may be abnormal

Prefibrotic Stage

- Mild anemia
- No or mild leukoerythroblastosis
- No or minimal poikilocytosis
- Mild to moderate leukocytosis
- Mild to marked thrombocytosis
- Hypercellular marrow
- Neutrophilic and megakaryocytic proliferation

Fibrotic Stage

- Leukoerythroblastosis
- Poikilocytosis
- Moderate to marked anemia
- Variable white blood cell count
- Variable platelet count
- Decreased marrow cellularity
- Increased marrow reticulin and collagen
- Megakaryocytic proliferation

Diagnostic Scheme

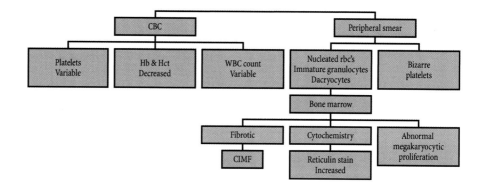

CHRONIC MYELOGENOUS LEUKEMIA

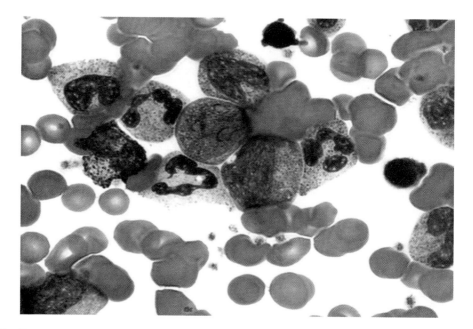

Figure IIB4-5   Peripheral blood smear.

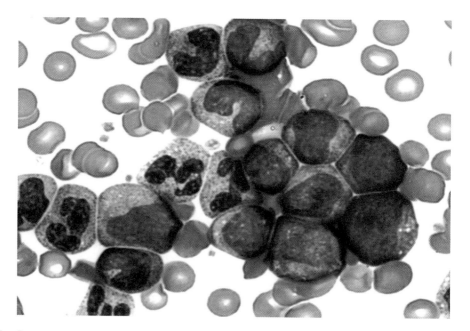

Figure IIB4-6   Bone marrow smear.

Clinical Features

- Occurs most frequently in middle-aged people—peak age 50–60 years
- Accounts for about 25% of adult leukemias
- Weight loss, night sweats, anorexia, visual disturbances, and bone pain
- Splenomegaly and hepatomegaly
- Anemia, bleeding disorders, and gout

Pathology

- Three stages
  - Chronic stable phase (CML-CP)
  - Accelerated phase (CML-AP)
  - Blastic phase (CML-BP)
- Normal bone marrow cells are replaced with cells containing an abnormal G-group chromosome called the Philadelphia or Ph chromosome (90–95% of cases)
- Translocation of material from the long arm of 22 to the long arm of 9 and from 9 to 22
  - Fuses the BCR gene from chromosome 22 with regions of the ABL gene on chromosome 9
- Double Philadelphia chromosome is associated with blastic transformation and accelerated phase

Laboratory Features

White Blood Cells

- Increased to $\geq 170 \times 10^9$/L
- Entire maturation series of granulocytes is seen but no toxic changes
- Eosinophilia
- Basophilia

Red Blood Cells

- Normocytic/normochromic anemia
- Occasional nucleated red blood cells

Platelets

- Typically increased but may be normal or decreased

Bone Marrow

- 90–100% cellularity
- M:E ratio 10:1–50:1
- Pseudo–Gaucher cells

Cytochemistry

- Leukocyte alkaline phosphatase level markedly decreased (score is usually ≤ 10)

Diagnostic Criteria (CML-CP)

Peripheral Blood

- Leukocytosis due to neutrophils in various stages of maturation
- Usually <2% blasts
- Basophilia
- <3% monocytes
- Normal or increased platelet count
- Mild anemia

Bone Marrow

- Hypercellular
- <5% blasts
- Smaller than normal megakaryocytes with hypolobulated nuclei
- Reticulin fibers increased
- Eosinophils may be increased
- Pseudo–Gaucher cells and sea-blue histiocytes may be seen

Diagnostic Criteria (CML-AP)

Peripheral Blood

- One or more of the following:
  - 10–19% myeloblasts
  - $\geq 20\%$ basophils
  - Platelet count $<100 \times 10^9/L$
  - Platelet count $>1000 \times 10^9/L$
  - Increasing numbers of white blood cells

Bone Marrow

■ One or more of the following:
  ■ 10–19% myeloblasts
  ■ Dysgranulopoiesis
  ■ Dysmegakaryopoiesis
  ■ Marked collagen or reticulin fibrosis

Diagnostic Criteria (CML-BP)

■ ≥20% blasts in blood or bone marrow
■ Extramedullary proliferation of blasts
■ Presence of large clusters of blasts in bone marrow

Diagnostic Scheme

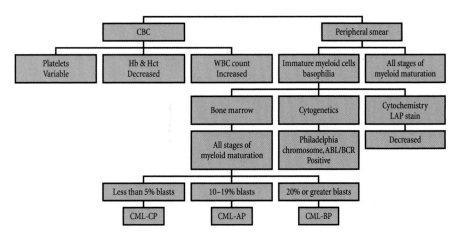

CHRONIC NEUTROPHILIC LEUKEMIA

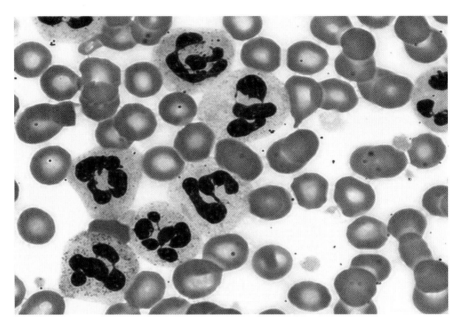

Figure IIB4-7   Peripheral blood smear.

Clinical Features

- Usually 50 years or older
- Equal gender distribution
- Splenomegaly
- Hepatomegaly

Pathology

- Very rare
- Seen with plasma dyscrasias
- Clonal disorder

Laboratory Features

White Blood Cells

- Persistent neutrophilia ($>25 \times 10^9$/L)
- Predominant cell is the neutrophil ($>80\%$) with a possible increase in bands
- $<1\%$ myeloblasts
- Monocytes $<1 \times 10^9$/L

Red Blood Cells

- Normocytic/normochromic anemia

Platelets

- Normal

Bone Marrow

- Granulocytic hypercellularity
- Myeloid:erythroid ratio about 5:1–25:1
- $<5\%$ myeloblasts
- No myelofibrosis

Cytochemistry

- Increased leukocyte alkaline phosphatase level

Cytogenetics

- Philadelphia chromosome negative

Diagnostic Scheme

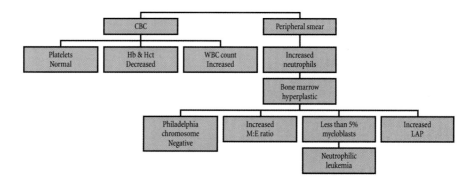

ESSENTIAL THROMBOCYTHEMIA

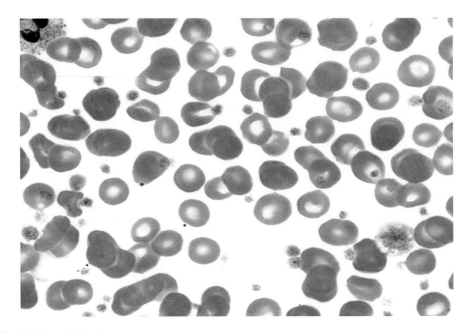

Figure **IIB4-8**   Peripheral blood smear.

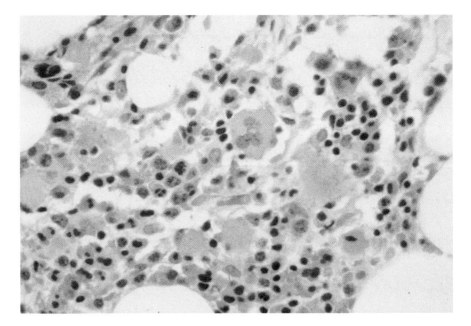

Figure **IIB4-9**   Bone marrow biopsy.

Clinical Features

- Also known as primary thrombocytosis or idiopathic thrombocytosis
- Patients are usually older than 50 years
- Splenomegaly
- Epistaxis, hemorrhage, or thrombosis

Pathology

- Clonal abnormality involving the megakaryocytic lineage
- Absence of Philadelphia chromosome
- No specific genetic or biologic markers—other causes for thrombocytosis must be excluded

Laboratory Features

White Blood Cells

- Usually normal or mildly increased
- Basophilia absent or minimal

Red Blood Cells

- Normocytic/normochromic anemia
- Microcytic, hypochromic anemia if there is gastrointestinal tract blood loss
- Red blood cell mass not elevated
- No dacryocytes or leukoerythroblastosis

Platelets

- Count $>600 \times 10^9/L$
- Aggregates
- Small to giant platelets

Bone Marrow

- Normocellular or slightly hypercellular
- Proliferation of large to giant megakaryocytes, bizarre forms seen
- Megakaryocyte mass increased
- Increased megakaryocytes arranged in clusters

Diagnostic Scheme

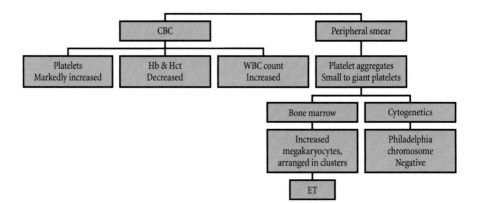

HYPEREOSINOPHILIC SYNDROME

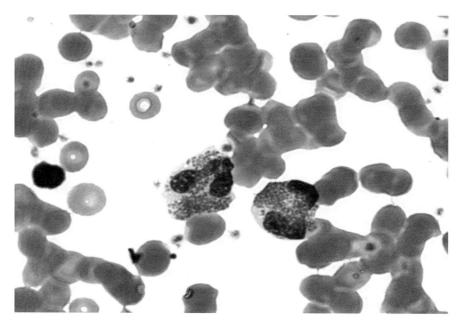

Figure IIB4-10   Peripheral blood smear.

Clinical Features

- Fever
- Weight loss
- Congestive heart failure
- Dyspnea
- More common in men than women

Pathology

- Absolute eosinophil count of $>1.5 \times 10^9$/L for 6 months or longer without clinical evidence of other known causes
- Cardiopulmonary dysfunction may be due to the excessive infiltration of mature eosinophils in multiple organs
- No evidence of eosinophil clonality

Laboratory Features

White Blood Cells

- Eosinophils increased
- Abnormal eosinophils
  - Vacuoles
  - Degranulation
  - Hypersegmentation or hyposegmentation

Red Blood Cells

- Decreased

Platelets

- Decreased

Diagnostic Scheme

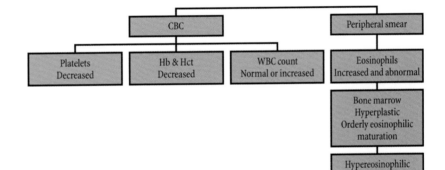

POLYCYTHEMIA VERA

Clinical Features

- Usually diagnosed in persons aged 55–70 years
- Slight male predominance
- Headache, confusion, altered mental status, dizziness, visual changes, tinnitus, and paresthesia
- Weight loss, epigastric pain, gout, pruritus, thrombosis, and hemorrhage
- Plethora, hypertension, and a mild to moderate degree of splenomegaly and hepatomegaly

Pathology

- Malignancy
- Excessive bone marrow production of the red blood cells and increase in total red blood cell volume
- White blood cell and platelet counts may also increase to a lesser extent
- Increased blood viscosity
- Thrombosis is a complication in more than half of the cases
- Myelofibrosis or acute myeloid leukemia may develop
- Polycythemic stage
  - Increased red blood cell mass
- "Spent" phase and post-polycythemic myelofibrosis and myeloid metaplasia
  - Anemia
  - Bone marrow fibrosis
  - Extramedullary hematopoiesis
  - Hypersplenism

Laboratory Features

White Blood Cells

- Increased count
- Immature forms usually not seen
- Eosinophils and basophils may be increased
- Leukocyte alkaline phosphatase level increased in three-quarters of cases

Red Blood Cells

- Hemoglobin level increased
- Hematocrit level increased
- Red blood cell mass increased

Platelets

■ Increased

Bone Marrow

■ Hyperplastic
■ Erythroid hyperplasia
■ Increased megakaryocytes
■ Granulocytic hyperplasia
■ Increased reticulin in post-polycythemic myelofibrosis and myeloid metaplasia
■ Iron stores are often depleted

Traditional Criteria for Diagnosis

Meet three major criteria or two major and two minor criteria

Major Criteria

■ Increased red blood cell mass
■ Splenomegaly
■ Normal oxygen level

Minor Criteria

■ Platelet count >400 × 10^9/L
■ White blood cell count >12.0 × 10^9/L
■ Elevated leukocyte alkaline phosphatase level
■ Elevated vitamin B_{12} level or unbound vitamin B_{12} binding capacity

Another Traditional Criteria for Diagnosis

Meet three major criteria or two major and two minor criteria

Major Criteria

■ Elevated red blood cell mass
■ Normal oxygen level
■ Splenomegaly

Minor Criteria

■ Thrombocytosis
■ Neutrophil leukocytosis
■ Positive endogenous erythroid colony assay or low serum erythropoietin level

World Health Organization Criteria for Diagnosis

Elevated red blood cell mass
No identified cause of secondary erythrocytosis
Plus one of the following:

■ Splenomegaly
■ Clonal abnormality, excluding Ph chromosome or BCR/ALB fusion gene
■ In vivo formation of endogenous erythroid colony

Or any two of the following:

■ Thrombocytosis $>400 \times 10^9$/L
■ White blood cell count $>12 \times 10^9$/L
■ Panmyelosis of the bone marrow with prominent erythroid and megakaryocytic proliferation
■ Low serum erythropoietin levels

Diagnostic Scheme

See Unit II, Section A, Chapter 1 Polycythemia Vera

CHAPTER

5

Myelodysplastic/ Myeloproliferative Diseases

ATYPICAL CHRONIC MYELOID LEUKEMIA

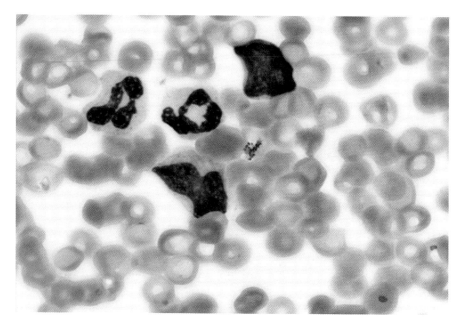

Figure **IIB5-1**   Peripheral blood smear.

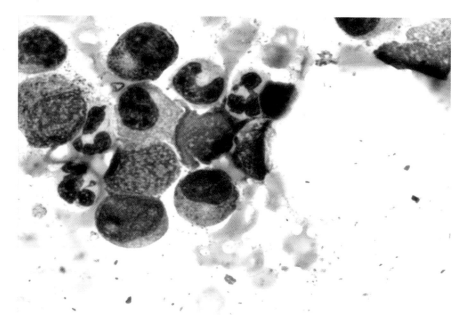

Figure **IIB5-2**   Bone marrow smear.

Clinical Features

- Occurs in about 1–2% of the chronic myelogenous leukemias
- Patients are usually elderly
- Fatigue, bleeding disorders
- Splenomegaly
- Hepatomegaly

Pathology

- Myelodysplastic as well as myeloproliferative features at the time of initial diagnosis
- Principal involvement of the granulocytic line
- No Philadelphia chromosome or BCR/ABL fusion gene
- No specific chromosomal abnormalities but may see +8, +13, del (20q), i (17q) del (12p)

Laboratory Features

White Blood Cells

- Leukocytosis is variable
- Immature and dysplastic
- >10% immature cells
- <20% blasts
- Minimal monocytosis but <10% relative monocytosis
- Basophilia not prominent
- Dysgranulopoiesis and pseudo–Pelger-Huët cells may be seen

Red Blood Cells

- Decreased number
- Dyserythropoiesis
- Macroovalocytosis

Platelets

- Decreased

Bone Marrow

- Hypercellular
- Granulopoiesis
- <20% blasts
- Dysgranulopoiesis
- Decreased megakaryocytes

Cytochemistry

- Leukocyte alkaline phosphatase level variable

Diagnostic Scheme

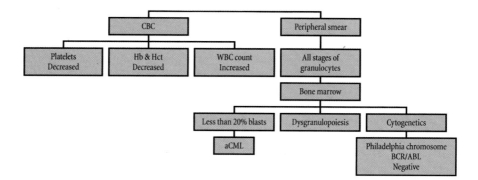

CHRONIC MYELOMONOCYTIC LEUKEMIA

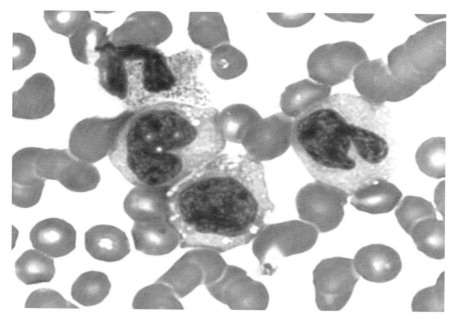

Figure IIB5-3   Peripheral blood smear.

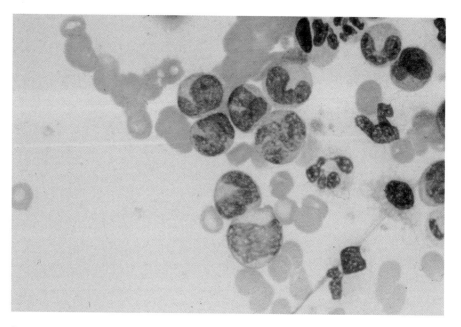

Figure IIB5-4   Bone marrow smear.

Clinical Features

- Occurs most commonly in persons older than 50 years
- Fatigue and weakness
- Hemorrhagic symptoms
- Infection is the most common cause of death
- Hepatomegaly and splenomegaly may be present, especially when the white blood cell count is elevated
- May have skin infiltrations

Pathology

- Expansion of abnormal cells in the bone marrow and a decrease in normal cells
- Rearrangements of genetic material may be important in the activation of proto-oncogenes to oncogenes
- Specific abnormalities have not been identified

Laboratory Features

White Blood Cells

- Usually normal to decreased
- <20% blasts
- >1 × 10^9/L monocytes
- May be neutropenia
- Dysgranulopoiesis
- Eosinophils and basophils are normal to decreased

Red Blood Cells

- Normocytic to macrocytic anemia
- Dimorphic population
- Nucleated red blood cells

Platelets

- Decreased count
- Abnormal forms may be found

Bone Marrow

- Usually hypercellular
- Granulocytic proliferation
- Slight dysgranulopoiesis
- Dyserythropoiesis
- Slight dysmegakaryopoiesis
- Increased monocytic precursors

Subcategories (World Health Organization)

CMML-1

- <5% blasts in blood
- <10% blasts in bone marrow

CMML-1 With Eosinophilia

- Previous criteria with an eosinophil count $>1.5 \times 10^9$/L

CMML-2

- 5–19% blasts in blood
- 10–19% blasts in bone marrow
- Or Auer rods present and <20% blasts in blood or bone marrow

CMML-2 With Eosinophilia

- Previous criteria with an eosinophil count $>1.5 \times 10^9$/L

Cytochemistry

- Nonspecific esterase positive
- Myeloperoxidase and Sudan black B negative or weakly positive
- Periodic acid–Schiff negative

Diagnostic Scheme

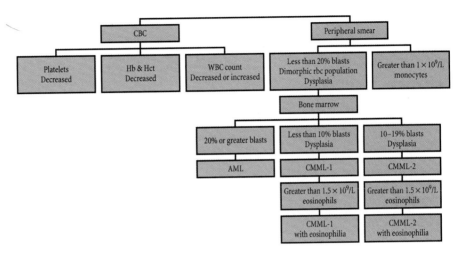

JUVENILE MYELOMONOCYTIC LEUKEMIA

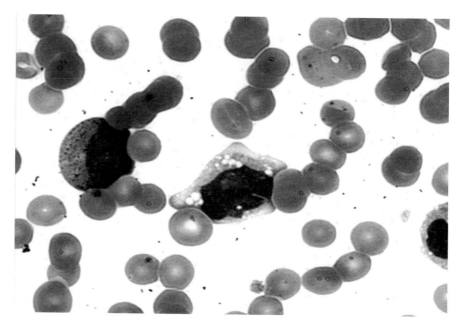

Figure IIB5-5   Peripheral blood smear.

Clinical Features

- Age of onset ranges from 1 month to early adolescence
- 2–3% of all leukemias in children
- 20–30% of all myelodysplastic and myeloproliferative diseases in children
- Approximately 75% of the cases occur in children younger than 3 years
- Malaise, pallor, fever, and recurrent infections
- Skin rashes
- Hepatosplenomegaly
- Leukemic infiltration of organs

Pathology

- May be a genetic predisposition
- Exact cause has not been elucidated
- No specific cytogenetic abnormalities
- No Philadelphia chromosome or BCR/ABL fusion gene

Laboratory Features

White Blood Cells

- Increased number
- Increase in all granulocytes
- Monocytosis
- <10% blasts and promonocytes
- Eosinophilia and basophilia not prominent

Red Blood Cells

- Nucleated red blood cells
- Normocytic/normochromic or macrocytic/normochromic anemia

Platelets

- Decreased

Bone Marrow

- Granulocytic hypercellularity
- 5–10% monocytes
- <20% blasts and promonocytes
- No Auer rods
- Dysgranulopoiesis
- Dyserythropoiesis
- Dysmegakaryopoiesis
- Decreased numbers of megakaryocytes

Cytochemistry

- Nonspecific esterase positive in monocytic precursors
- Leukocyte alkaline phosphatase stain may be decreased

Diagnostic Criteria (World Health Organization)

- Peripheral monocytosis ($>1 \times 10^9$/L)
- <30% blasts and promonocytes
- Philadelphia chromosome and BCR/ABL fusion gene negative
- Plus two or more of the following:
  - Increased hemoglobin F (for age)
  - Immature granulocytes in blood
  - White blood cell count $>10 \times 10^9$/L
  - Clonal chromosomal abnormalities
  - In vitro granulocyte-macrophage colony-stimulating factor hypersensitivity of myeloid progenitors

Diagnostic Scheme

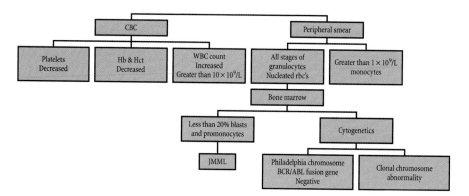

CHAPTER

6

Chronic Lymphoproliferative Disorders

ADULT T-CELL LYMPHOMA LEUKEMIA

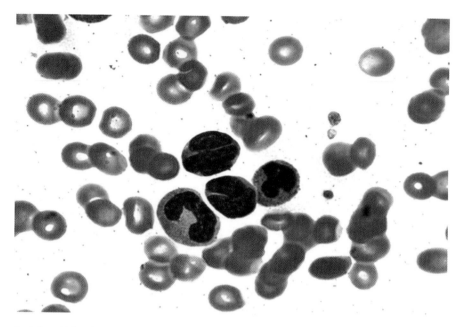

Figure IIB6-1   Peripheral blood smear.

Clinical Features

- Evolves rapidly
- Skin lesions
- Hepatosplenomegaly
- Adenopathy

Pathology

- Only chronic leukemia where the virus has been demonstrated (human T-cell lymphotrophic virus type I)
- Invasion of cells by the virus causes cell proliferation
- Rearrangement of T cell receptor (TCR) genes
- CD4, CD25 positive and terminal deoxynucleotidyl trasnferase negative

Laboratory Features

White Blood Cells

- May be only a few abnormal cells in the peripheral blood
- Cells have highly convoluted nuclei with deep multilobulated indentation
- Cell size and N/C ratio is larger than that of normal lymphocytes

Red Blood Cells

- Normocytic/normochromic anemia

Platelets

- Normal to decreased

Bone Marrow

- Presence of infiltrates and evidence of bony remodeling and fibrosis

Diagnostic Scheme

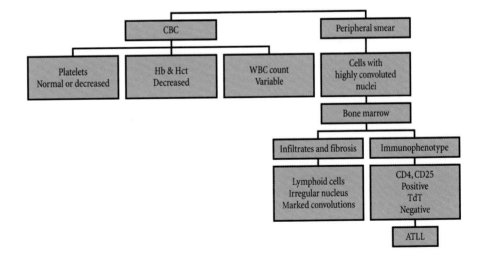

CHRONIC LYMPHOCYTIC LEUKEMIA

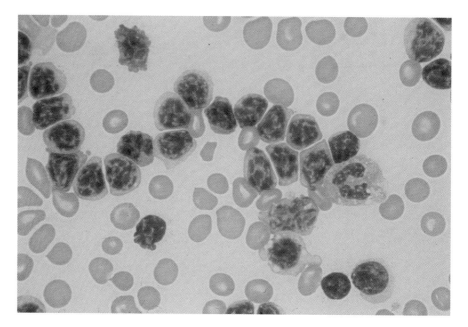

Peripheral blood smear.

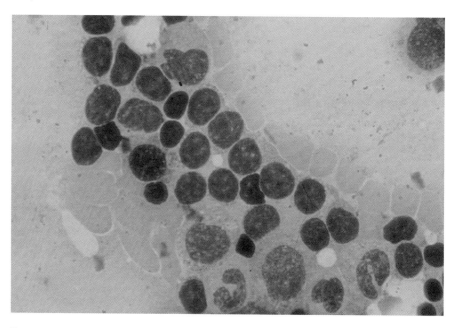

Bone marrow smear.

Clinical Features

- Occurs most frequently in persons older than 50 years and accounts for about 30% of leukemias
- Enlargement of superficial lymph nodes is common
- With disease progression, splenomegaly and hepatomegaly develop
- Infections are frequent
- May develop a secondary warm autoimmune hemolytic anemia
- Some patients are asymptomatic

Pathology

- Proliferation and accumulation of B lymphocytes
- Monoclonal B-cell population with low-density surface immunoglobulin
- Chromosomal abnormalities
  - Trisomy 12 is most common and associated with poorer prognosis
  - 14q+, 13q+, and 11q+
  - Deletion of chromosome 6
- Approximately 3.5% of chronic lymphocytic leukemia cases transform into a more aggressive stage with the formation of a mass of high-grade large-cell lymphoma cells

Laboratory Features

White Blood Cells

- Increased to $20–200 \times 10^9$/L
- Absolute lymphocytosis
- Typical, small lymphocytes, with a hypermature-appearing nucleus
- Smudge cells present
- <10% prolymphocytes
- Larger cells may be seen in Richter's syndrome

Red Blood Cells

- Normocytic/normochromic anemia

Platelets

- Normal
- Often decreased with disease progression

Bone Marrow

- Replacement by lymphocytes
- ≤10% prolymphocytes

Immunophenotype

- CD5, CD19, CD23, and CD79a positive
- CD20 and sIg weak

Prognostic Scheme

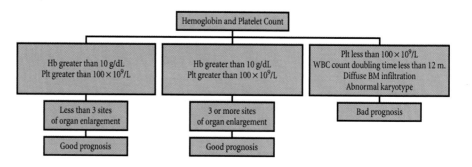

Diagnostic Scheme

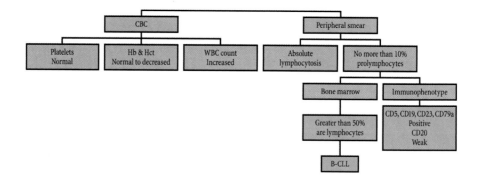

HAIRY CELL LEUKEMIA

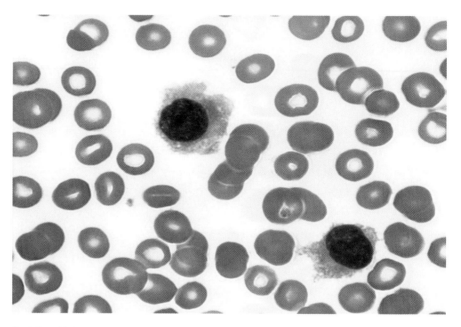

Figure IIB6-4   Peripheral blood smear.

Clinical Features

- Male predominance (5:1)
- Median age of onset is about 50 years
- Weakness and fatigue
- Easy bruising and bleeding tendency
- Recurrent infections
- Hepatomegaly and splenomegaly

Pathology

- Usually a B-cell disease
- T cells are involved in <1% of cases

Laboratory Features

White Blood Cells

- Increased
- Presence of hairy lymphocytes
- Neutropenia

Red Blood Cells

- Moderate normocytic/normochromic anemia

Platelets

- $<100 \times 10^9$/L in 50% of patients

Bone Marrow

- Cannot be aspirated in more than half of the cases because of reticulin fibers

Cytochemistry

- Tartrate-resistant acid phosphatase positive
- Specific esterase (naphthol AS-D chloroacetate esterase) and myeloperoxidase reactions are negative

Immunophenotype

- CD103, CD20, CD19, CD22, CD11c, CD25, FMC7, and sIg positive

Diagnostic Scheme

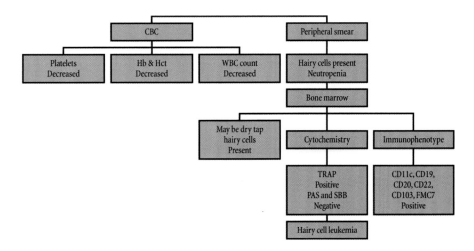

LARGE GRANULAR LYMPHOCYTIC LEUKEMIA

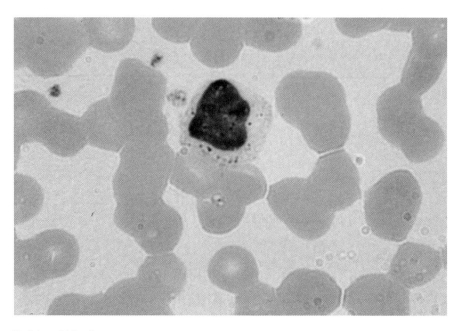

Figure IIB6-5   Peripheral blood smear.

Clinical Features

- Large granular lymphocytes are killer cells that differentiate into natural killer and T-cell types
- Clonal diseases may arise from either of the two large granular lymphocyte lineages: T-large granular lymphocytic leukemia (T-LGL) and natural killer-large granular (NK-LGL) lymphocytic leukemia

T-LGL

- Patients are usually older than 50 years
- Some patients are asymptomatic
- Recurrent infections
- Persistent neutropenia and lymphocytosis
- Rheumatoid arthritis
- Splenomegaly

NK-LGL

- Not as common as T-LGL
- Occurs in a younger group of patients
- Aggressive malignancy
- Fever, weight loss, and night sweats
- Marked hepatosplenomegaly and lymphadenopathy
- Multiorgan failure

Pathology

- Defects in programmed cell death
- Viral infections may be an initial stimulus
- Neutropenia in T-LGL is related to antineutrophil antibodies or circulating immune complexes

Laboratory Features

T-LGL

White Blood Cells

- Lymphocytosis in the range of $4.0–10.0 \times 10^9/L$
- Presence of large granular lymphocytes
    - CD3 and CD8 positive

Red Blood Cells

- May have a macrocytic anemia

Platelets

- Normal to decreased

Bone Marrow

- Lymphocytic infiltration

NK-LGL

White Blood Cells

- High lymphocyte counts
- NK-LGLs predominate
    - CD3 negative
    - CD56 positive

Red Blood Cells

- Normocytic/normochromic anemia

Platelets

- Decreased

Diagnostic Scheme

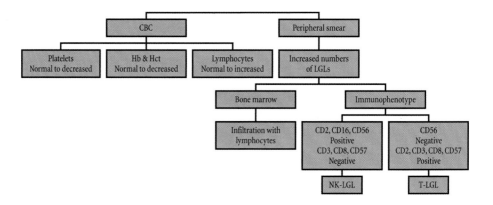

PROLYMPHOCYTIC LEUKEMIA

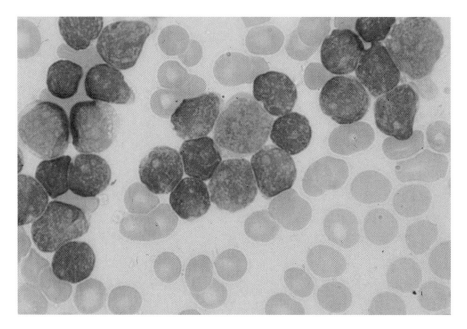

Figure IIB6-6   Peripheral blood smear.

Clinical Features

- Median age of occurrence is 60 years, with a male predominance
- Systemic symptoms such as weakness, fatigue, weight loss, fever, and possibly abdominal pain are seen
- Absent or minimal lymphadenopathy
- Massive splenomegaly, hepatomegaly, and bone marrow infiltration

Pathology

- Disease of the B (>80%) or T cells
- T-cell disease is more aggressive and has a higher incidence of adenopathy, leukocytosis, skin infiltration, and hepatomegaly
- Exhibit heavy and light chain Ig gene rearrangements
- Cells express much more sIg than do chronic lymphocytic leukemia cells
- Chromosomal abnormalities
  - B-PLL
    - 14 q+
  - T-PLL
    - Inv (14)

Laboratory Features

White Blood Cells

- Typically $>100 \times 10^9/L$
- $>55\%$ prolymphocytes
- Cells contain a large, vesicular nucleolus, condensed nuclear chromatin and may have moderate cytoplasmic basophilia
- T cells have nuclear irregularities

Red Blood Cells

- Normocytic/normochromic anemia

Platelets

- Decreased

Cytochemistry

- T-PLL demonstrates focal positivity with acid phosphatase

Immunophenotype (B-Cell Type)

- CD19, CD20, CD22, CD79a and b, FMC7, and sIg positive
- CD5 positive in less than one-third of cases
- CD23 negative

Diagnostic Scheme

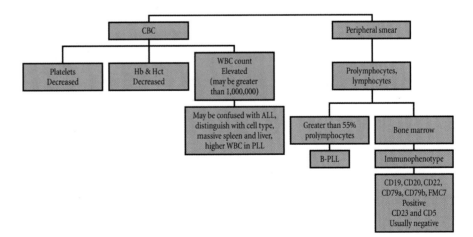

SÉZARY SYNDROME

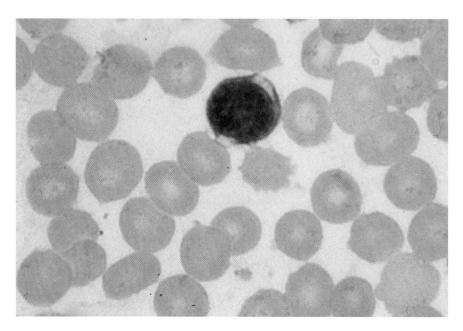

Peripheral blood smear.

Clinical Features

- Generalized erythroderma
- Pruritus
- Infections
- Uncommon malignancy seen more commonly in males (2:1)
- Median age of occurrence is 55 years

Pathology

- Systemic phase of cutaneous T-cell lymphoma
- Malignant proliferation of T lymphocytes
- Many structural and numerical alterations but no specific abnormalities are associated

Laboratory Features

White Blood Cells

- Hyperconvoluted lymphoid cells in blood

Red Blood Cells

■ May have a normocytic/normochromic anemia

Platelets

■ Normal to decreased

Bone Marrow

■ Eosinophilia
■ Monocytosis
■ Plasmacytosis
■ Rare infiltrates of Sézary cells

Cytochemistry

■ Focal positivity with acid phosphatase
■ Peroxidase, alkaline phosphatase, and specific esterase (chloroacetate esterase) negative

Immunophenotype

■ CD2, CD3, CD4, CD5, and TCR beta positive
■ CD7 and CD8 negative

Chemistry

■ IgE and IgA increased

Diagnostic Scheme

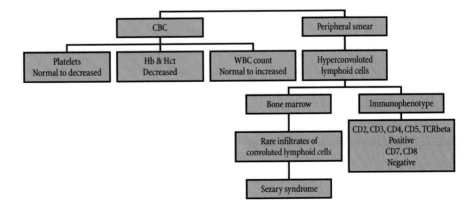

CHAPTER

7

Lymphomas

HODGKIN LYMPHOMA

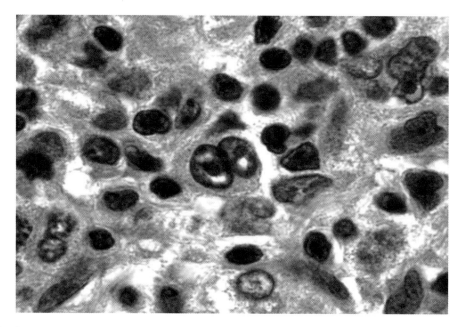

Figure **IIB7-1**   Lymph node biopsy.

Clinical Features

- More common in males than in females
- Peak incidence is about the third decade of life
- Painless lymph node enlargement
- Cough and chest discomfort
- Drenching sweats at night, fever, and weight loss

Pathology

- Malignant cells probably originate from follicular center B cells

Laboratory Features

White Blood Cells

- Variable, may be elevated in about 25% of cases
- May have slight eosinophilia

Red Blood Cells

- Anemia is rare

Platelets

- Thrombocytopenia is rare

Bone Marrow

- Recommended for staging
- Bone marrow infiltration is a serious manifestation

Immunophenotype

- CD20, CD30, and CD15 positive and most useful markers

Lymph Node Biopsy

- A large, intact lymph node is examined for the presence of Reed-Sternberg cells
  - Giant cells with large, eosinophilic, inclusion-like nucleoli; a thick, well-defined nuclear membrane; and pale-staining chromatin
  - The classic cell has two-mirror image nuclei

Diagnostic Scheme

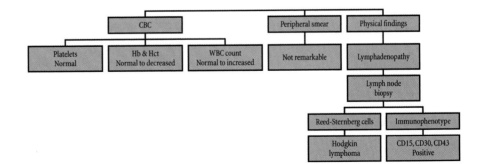

NON-HODGKIN'S LYMPHOMAS OF B-CELL ORIGIN—DIFFUSE LARGE B-CELL LYMPHOMA

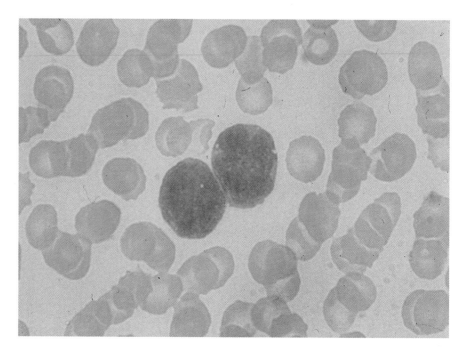

Figure IIB7-2   Peripheral blood smear.

Clinical Features

■ Usually occurs in older males
■ Adenopathy
■ Hepatosplenomegaly

Pathology

■ Chromosomal abnormalities may be observed
■ Oncogenes may be implicated
■ May be associated with viral infections
■ Lymphoid antigens present
　■ B cell—CD19, CD20, CD22, and others
■ 40% of all cases

Laboratory Features

Cell Type

- Sheets of large heterogeneous lymphocytes with variable cytoplasm

Immunophenotype

- CD19, CD20, and CD43 positive
- CD10, bcl-2 plus/minus

Diagnostic Scheme

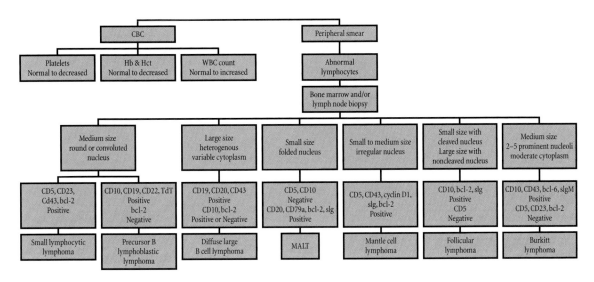

NON-HODGKIN'S LYMPHOMAS OF B-CELL ORIGIN—PRECURSOR B-LYMPHOBLASTIC LEUKEMIA/LYMPHOMA

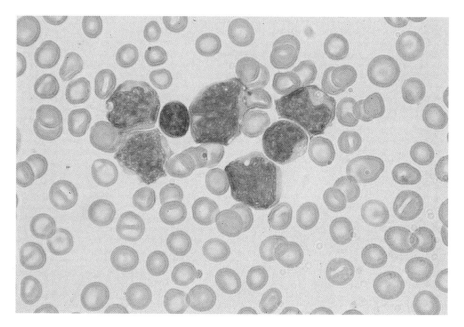

Figure IIB7-3   Peripheral blood smear.

Clinical Features

■ Most common in children
■ Adenopathy

Pathology

■ Chromosomal abnormalities may be observed, some relate to prognosis
■ Oncogenes may be implicated
■ Lymphoid antigens present
    ■ B cell—most CD10 positive, CD19, CD20, CD22
■ Highly aggressive but curable

Laboratory Findings

Cell Type

- Medium size
- Round or convoluted nucleus
- Fine chromatin
- Scant cytoplasm

Immunophenotype

- CD10 (most but not all positive), CD19, CD22, TdT positive (rarely negative)
- CD20 and CD24 (usually positive)
- CD13 and CD33 negative (rarely positive)
- bcl-2, sIg negative

Diagnostic Scheme

(see NON-HODGKIN'S LYMPHOMAS OF B-CELL ORIGIN—DIFFUSE LARGE
   B-CELL LYMPHOMA)

NON-HODGKIN'S LYMPHOMAS OF B-CELL ORIGIN—SMALL LYMPHOCYTIC LYMPHOMA OR CHRONIC LYMPHOCYTIC LEUKEMIA

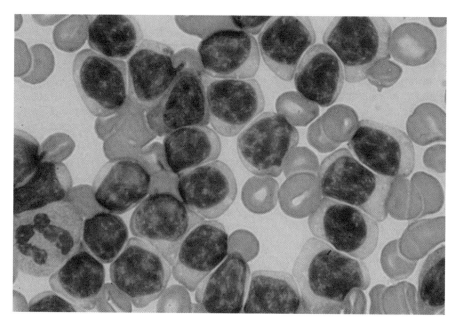

Figure IIB7-4   Peripheral blood smear.

Clinical Features

■ Usually occurs in older males
■ Adenopathy
■ Hepatosplenomegaly fairly common

Pathology

■ Chromosomal abnormalities may be observed
■ Oncogenes may be implicated
■ Lymphoid antigens present
   ■ B cell—CD19, CD20, and CD22
■ Neoplasm of a small B cell
■ Indolent disease
■ May show prolymphocytoid transformation
■ Complication by large-cell lymphoma can occur (Richter's syndrome)
■ Older patients present with diffuse adenopathy, splenic disease, and marrow involvement

Laboratory Features

Cell Types

- Small B cell
- Round nucleus
- Coarse chromatin
- Scanty pale-staining cytoplasm

Immunophenotype

- sIg, CD5, CD20, CD23, CD43, and bcl-2 positive
- cIg and CD10 negative

Cytogenetics

- Trisomy 12
- t(14;19)
- 13q and 14q abnormalities

Diagnostic Scheme

(see NON-HODGKIN'S LYMPHOMAS OF B-CELL ORIGIN—DIFFUSE LARGE
B-CELL LYMPHOMA)

NON-HODGKIN'S LYMPHOMAS OF B-CELL ORIGIN—MUCOSA-ASSOCIATED LYMPHOID TISSUE LYMPHOMA

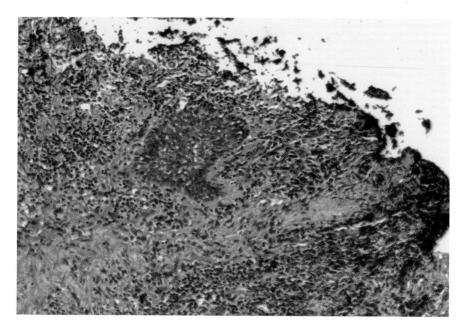

Figure IIB7-5   Tissue section.

Clinical Features

■ Occurs in extranodal sites such as the stomach, salivary glands, and thyroid

Pathology

■ Chromosomal abnormalities may be observed
■ Oncogenes may be implicated
■ Lymphoid antigens present
    ■ B cell—CD19, CD20, and CD22
■ Malignant cells arise from the B cells localized in the marginal zone of the follicle
■ Tend to be indolent and remain localized for long periods
■ Gastric MALT may be associated with *Helicobacter pylori* infections
■ Female predominance

Laboratory Findings

Cell Types

- Variable-sized lymphocytes
- Centrocytelike cells
- Monocytoid B cells

Immunophenotype

- CD20, CD 79a, bcl-2, sIg, some cIg positive
- CD5 and CD10 negative
- CD23 negative

Diagnostic Scheme

(see NON-HODGKIN'S LYMPHOMAS OF B-CELL ORIGIN—DIFFUSE LARGE
B-CELL LYMPHOMA)

NON-HODGKIN'S LYMPHOMAS OF B-CELL ORIGIN—MANTLE CELL LYMPHOMA (INTERMEDIATE LYMPHOCYTIC LYMPHOMA)

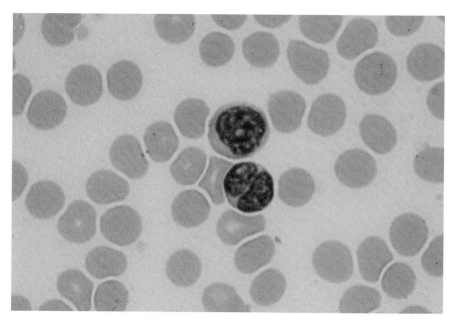

Figure IIB7-6   Peripheral blood smear.

Clinical Features

- Usually occurs in older males
- Adenopathy

Pathology

- Oncogenes may be implicated
- Lymphoid antigens present
  - B cell—CD19, CD20, and CD22
- Arises from the mantle cell of primary and secondary lymph node follicles
- Chromosomal abnormalities
  - t(11;14)
  - Rearranged bcl-1 gene
- Moderately aggressive

Laboratory Findings

Cell Type

- Small- to medium-sized cell
- Irregular nucleus
- Scant cytoplasm

Immunophenotype

- CD43, cyclin D1, sIg, CD5, bcl-2 positive
- cIg, CD10, and CD23 negative

Diagnostic Scheme

(see NON-HODGKIN'S LYMPHOMAS OF B-CELL ORIGIN—DIFFUSE LARGE
   B-CELL LYMPHOMA)

NON-HODGKIN'S LYMPHOMAS OF B-CELL ORIGIN—FOLLICULAR LYMPHOMAS

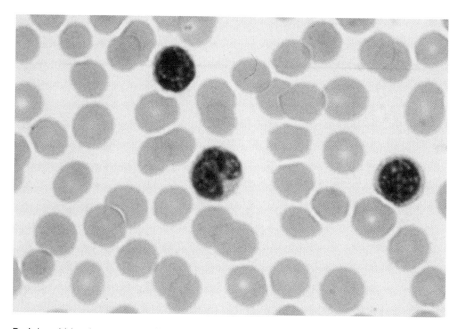

Peripheral blood smear—small follicular cell.

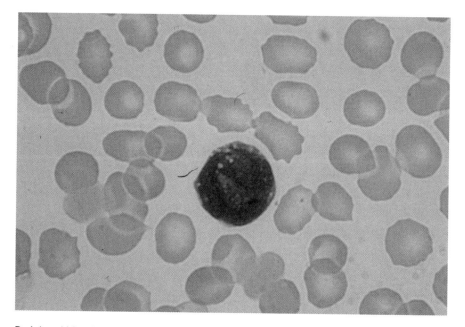

Peripheral blood smear—large follicular cell.

Clinical Features

- Usually occurs in older males
- Adenopathy

Pathology

- Oncogenes may be implicated
- Lymphoid antigens present
    - B cell—CD19, CD20, and CD22
- Arises from the follicular structure
- Chromosomal abnormalities
    - t(14;18)
    - Rearranged bcl-2 gene
        - bcl-2 oncogene prevents programmed cell death
- Indolent course

Laboratory Findings

Cell Types

- Based on origin of the malignancy in the follicle
    - Small cleaved follicle center cell (centrocytes)
        - Scant cytoplasm
    - Large follicle center cell (centroblasts)
        - Basophilic cytoplasm
    - Follicular pattern

Immunophenotype

- bcl-2, CD10, CD20, and sIg positive
- CD23+/−
- CD5 negative

Diagnostic Scheme

(see NON-HODGKIN'S LYMPHOMAS OF B-CELL ORIGIN—DIFFUSE LARGE
  B-CELL LYMPHOMA)

NON-HODGKIN'S LYMPHOMAS OF B-CELL ORIGIN—BURKITT'S LYMPHOMA

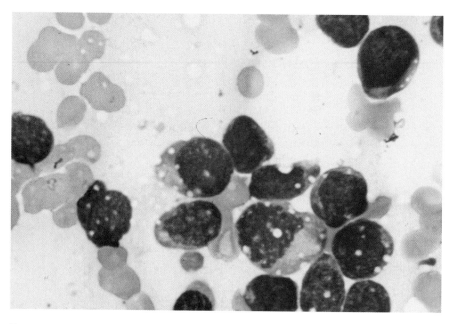

Figure IIB7-9   Bone marrow smear.

Clinical Features

- Usually occurs in children or young adults
- Adenopathy, but may have extranodal involvement
- Rapidly growing mass may be present, especially in the jaw bone

Pathology

- Oncogenes may be implicated
- Viruses such as Epstein-Barr virus and HIV may be associated
- Lymphoid antigens present
    - B cell—CD19, CD20, and CD22
- Diffuse, not follicular, lymphoma
- Undifferentiated B cells of unknown origin
- Highly aggressive
- Chromosomal abnormalities
    - IgH and IgL genes rearranged
    - t(8;14)

Laboratory Findings

Cell Types

- Monomorphic medium-sized cell
- Round nucleus
- 2–5 prominent nucleoli
- Moderate basophilic cytoplasm

Immunophenotype

- sIgM, CD10, CD43, and bcl-6 positive
- CD5, CD23, bcl-2 negative

Diagnostic Scheme

(see NON-HODGKIN'S LYMPHOMAS OF B-CELL ORIGIN—DIFFUSE LARGE B-CELL LYMPHOMA)

CHAPTER

8

Plasma Cell Disorders

PLASMA CELL LEUKEMIA

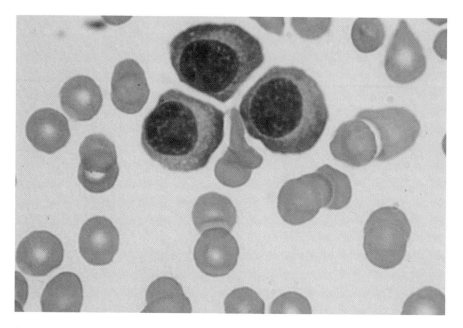

Figure **IIB8-1**   Peripheral blood smear.

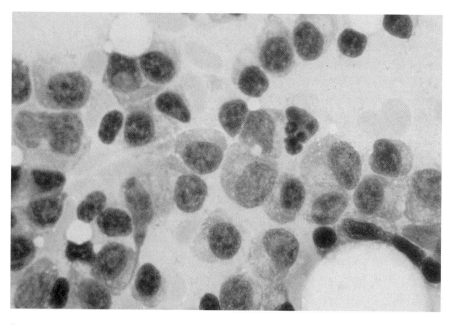

Figure **IIB8-2**   Bone marrow smear.

Clinical Features

- Hepatosplenomegaly
- Lymphadenopathy
- Lytic bone lesions are frequently present
- Severe anemia

Pathology

- Primary plasma cell leukemia demonstrates circulating myeloma cells at the time of diagnosis
- Secondary plasma cell leukemia represents the advanced stage of myeloma (a leukemic phase), which occurs as a terminal event in about 1–5% of cases

Laboratory Features

White Blood Cells

- Plasma cells in the peripheral blood (>20%)
- Leukocytosis

Red Blood Cells

- Severe normocytic/normochromic anemia
- Rouleaux

Platelets

- Decreased

Bone Marrow

- Diffuse plasma cell infiltration (50–100% of cells are plasma cells)
- Plasma cells are well differentiated
- Binucleated plasma cells may be present

Immunophenotype

- CD38, CD138 positive

Chemistries

- Increased serum calcium
- Increased blood urea nitrogen level
- Increased creatinine level

Diagnostic Scheme

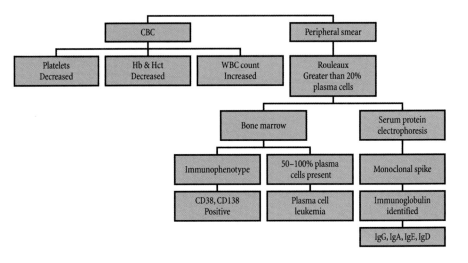

PLASMA CELL MYELOMA (MULTIPLE MYELOMA)

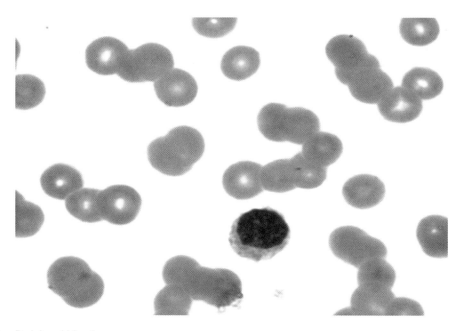

Figure **IIB8-3**   Peripheral blood smear.

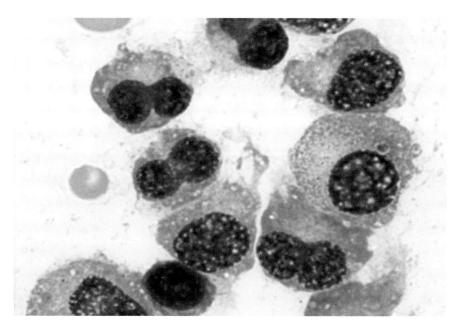

Figure **IIB8-4**   Bone marrow smear.

Clinical Features

- Fatigue
- Generalized aching
- Bone pain
- Lytic bone lesions
- Neurologic abnormalities
- Median age of onset is about 65 years
- Infections
- Renal failure

Pathology

- Malignant proliferation of a clone of plasma cells
- Plasma cells secrete complete or incomplete monoclonal immunoglobulins
- Prolonged excretion of Bence Jones protein in the urine often results in renal failure
- Increased susceptibility to infections

Laboratory Features

White Blood Cells

- Count is usually normal
- Plasma cells may be present

Red Blood Cells

- Normocytic/normochromic anemia
- Rouleaux
- Increased sedimentation rate

Platelets

- Normal to decreased
- Abnormal function

Bone Marrow

- Marrow plasmacytosis ($>10\%$)
- Myeloma cells are present
    - Single eccentrically placed nucleus
    - Nucleoli may be seen in finely divided chromatin
    - Various types of inclusions may be present

Immunophenotype

■ CD38, CD56, CD58, and CD138 positive

Chemistries

■ Serum and urine monoclonal protein
■ IgG, IgA, IgE, or IgD increased
■ Total protein increased

Diagnostic Scheme

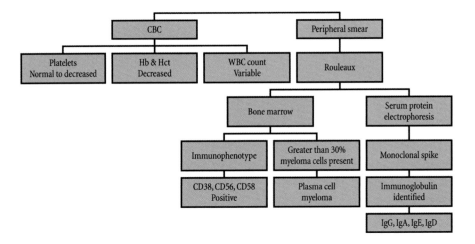

WALDENSTRÖM´S MACROGLOBINEMIA

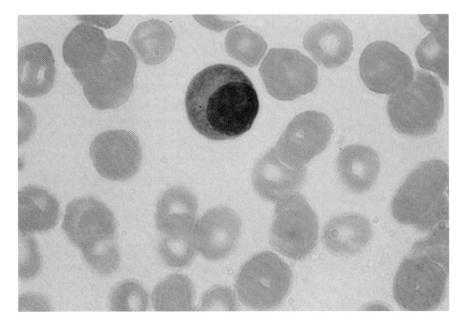

Figure **IIB8-5**   Peripheral blood smear.

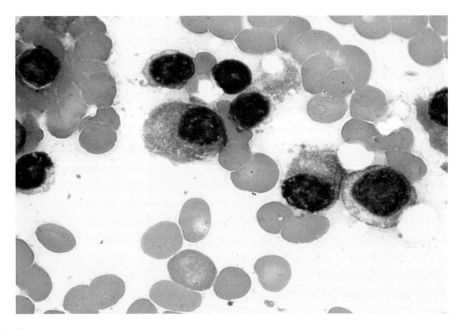

Figure **IIB8-6**   Bone marrow smear.

Clinical Features

- Usually occurs during the sixth and seventh decades of life
- More frequent in males than females
- Weakness and weight loss
- Progresses to hepatosplenomegaly and lymphadenopathy
- Bone pain is not prominent
- Headache, dizziness, and vertigo
- Recurrent infections
- Congestive heart failure
- Bleeding diathesis

Pathology

- Neoplasm arising from plasma cells and lymphoid cell populations
- Malignant clone is responsible for the synthesis of immunoglobulins containing the μ heavy chain
- Hyperviscosity may produce circulatory disturbances

Laboratory Features

White Blood Cells

- Normal or increased

Red Blood Cells

- Normocytic/normochromic anemia
- Rouleaux
- Increased sedimentation rate

Platelets

- Normal to decreased
- Abnormal function

Bone Marrow

- May result in a dry tap
- Large numbers of lymphoid cells

Chemistries

- Presence of Bence Jones protein in the urine in about one-quarter of cases
- Increased levels of IgM
- Increased levels of serum protein

Diagnostic Scheme

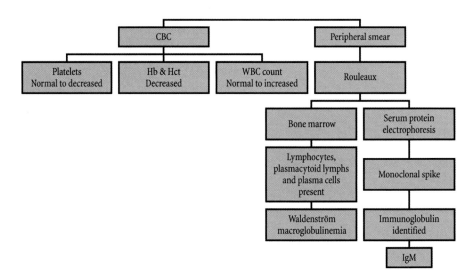

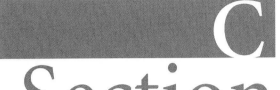

Section C

Miscellaneous Disorders

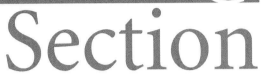

CHAPTER 1

Quantitative Platelet Disorders

THROMBOCYTOPENIA

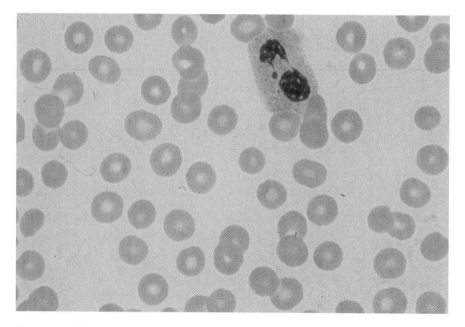

Figure **IIC1-1** Peripheral blood smear.

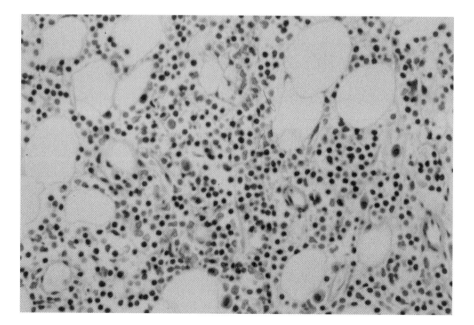

Figure **IIC1-2** Bone marrow biopsy.

Clinical Features

- Petechiae and purpura
- Mild to moderate mucosal bleeding
- Gingival bleeding

Pathology

- Decreased megakaryocytopoiesis
  - Congenital
  - Acquired
    - Marrow damage
    - Marrow infiltration
- Ineffective production
  - Congenital
    - May-Hegglin anomaly
    - Wiscott-Aldrich syndrome
  - Acquired
    - Vitamin B_{12} or folate deficiency
- Sequestration or dilutional
  - Hypersplenism
  - Massive transfusion
- Increased destruction
  - Nonimmune
    - Consumption
    - Disseminated intravascular coagulation, thrombotic thrombocytopenic purpura, hemolytic uremic syndrome, vasculitis
  - Immune
    - Idiopathic thrombocytopenic purpura
      - Acute
      - Chronic

Laboratory Features

White Blood Cells

- Varies with etiology

Red Blood Cells

- Varies with etiology

Platelets

- Decreased

Bone Marrow

■ Increased, normal, or decreased megakaryocytes

Diagnostic Scheme

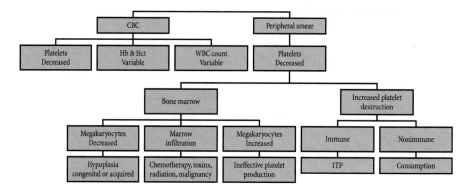

THROMBOCYTOSIS

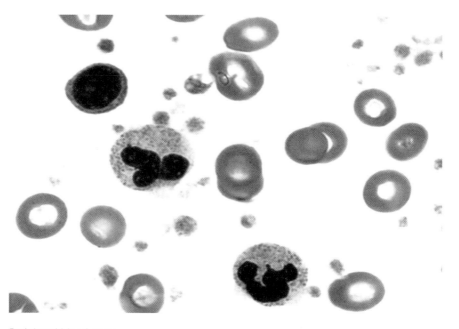

Figure **IIC1-3**   Peripheral blood smear.

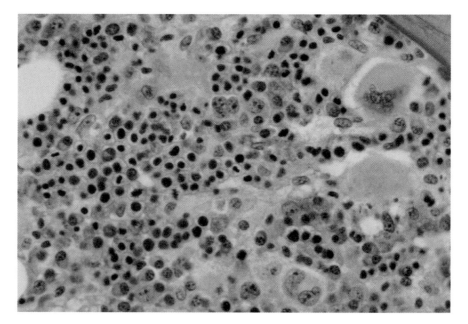

Figure **IIC1-4**   Bone marrow biopsy.

Clinical Features

- Reactive thrombocytosis is usually asymptomatic
- Autonomous thrombocytosis may be associated with bleeding and/or thrombosis

Pathology

- Secondary reactive thrombocytosis is associated with
  - Acute hemorrhage
  - Chronic inflammatory disorders
  - Hemolytic anemia
  - Severe iron deficiency
- Essential or primary thrombocythemia is associated with
  - Essential thrombocytosis
  - Other myeloproliferative diseases

Laboratory Features

White Blood Cells

- Varies with etiology

Red Blood Cells

- Varies with etiology

Platelets

Secondary Thrombocytosis

- Platelets increased
- Megakaryocytes increased
- Mean platelet volume is decreased or increased

Primary or Essential Thrombocytosis

- Platelets greatly increased
- Megakaryocytes increased
- Mean platelet volume is increased (chronic myelogenous leukemia, chronic idiopathic myelofibrosis)
- Mean platelet volume is normal (essential thrombocythemia, polycythemia vera)

Diagnostic Scheme

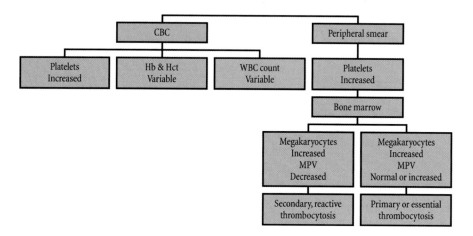

CHAPTER

2

Hematologic Disease Associated With Microorganisms

BABESIOSIS

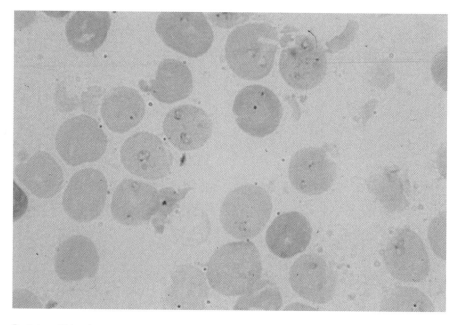

Figure II2-1   Peripheral blood smear.

Clinical Features

- May be asymptomatic from many months to years
- Malaise, fever, chills, fatigue, myalgia, and arthralgia
- Hepatosplenomegaly with jaundice
- Some fatalities have been reported

Pathology

- Rodents are the main reservoir, but some human infections with cattle and dog species of *Babesia* have been reported
- *Babesia* are major pathogens in wild and domestic animals that nearly destroyed the American cattle industry during the late nineteenth century
- Human infections are still rare and have similar epidemiology to Lyme disease but are less widely spread
- Transmitted by the bite of the deer tick but can be transmitted transplacentally and by blood transfusion

Laboratory Features

White Blood Cells

- Mild neutropenia

Red Blood Cells

- Mild to severe hemolytic anemia

Platelets

- Thrombocytopenia may occur
- *Babesia* organisms found on the blood smear
- Intraerythrocytic ring-shaped or pleomorphic parasites (piroplasms)
- Extraerythrocytic parasites found
- Unlike malaria, there is no pigment

Diagnostic Scheme

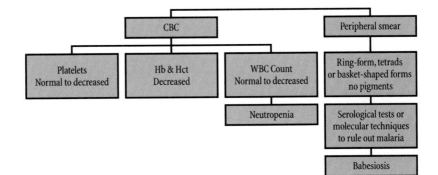

BORRELIOSIS

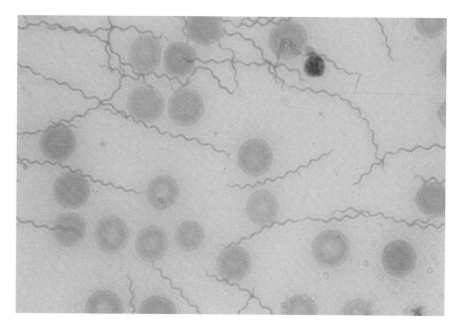

Figure II2-2   Peripheral blood smear.

Clinical Features

- High fever, shaking chills, delirium, headache, and muscle aches
- Cyclical pattern of symptoms corresponds to parasite development
- Pain in bones and joints
- Hepatosplenomegaly with tenderness
- Jaundice

Pathology

- Several species of *Borrelia* spirochetes
- Enter the body through the bite of a tick or through contamination of abraded skin with materials from crushed body lice

Laboratory Features

White Blood Cells

- Leukocytosis
- Neutrophilia

Red Blood Cells

- Not remarkable

Platelets

- Not remarkable

Presence of Spirochetes in Blood During a Febrile Episode

- Thin, undulant, and overtly spiral organisms
- Located between red blood cells

Diagnostic Scheme

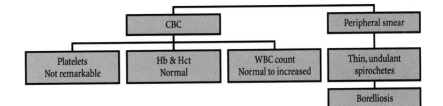

CANDIDIASIS

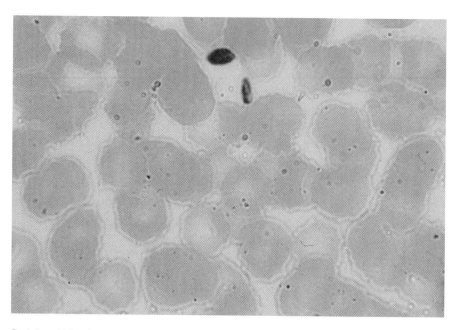

Figure II2-3   Peripheral blood smear.

Clinical Features

- Dysphagia, cough, itching, and burning
- Discharge—depends on primary location of infection
- Fever, chills, and headache
- May include shock, renal shutdown, and disseminated intravascular coagulation

Pathology

- Species of *Candida*, which are commensal organisms
- *Candida albicans* is the most common agent
- Immunocompromised people are at risk for infection
- Persons treated with broad-spectrum antibiotics and corticosteroids are at risk

Laboratory Features

White Blood Cells

- Leukocytosis

Red Blood Cells

- Anemia develops in severe infections

Platelets

- Thrombocytopenia may develop

Budding Yeast With Pseudo or True Hyphae Can Be Observed in the Blood

Diagnostic Scheme

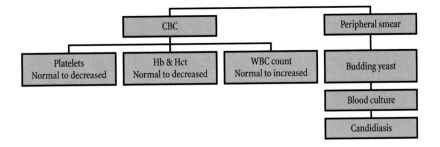

FILARIASIS

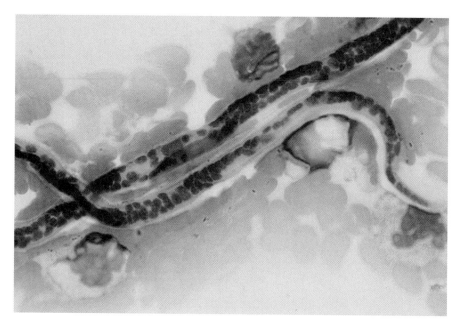

Peripheral blood smear.

Clinical Features

- Tissue-dwelling nematodes producing larvae that appear in blood, skin, and serous fluids
- May be asymptomatic
- Lymphadenitis to disruption of lymphatic vessels or drainage of lymph fluid
- Low-grade fever
- Maculopapular rash
- Urticaria

Pathology

- May be caused by *Wuchereria bancrofti, Brugia malayi, Brugia timori,* or *Loa Loa*
- Spread by mosquitoes or tabanid fly when infective larvae escape from the mosquito, enter the puncture wound, and migrate to the lymphatics
- Adult worms develop in the lymphatics
- Gravid females produce microfilariae that circulate in blood
- Bancroftian filariasis present in tropical areas of Africa, Asia, the Pacific, and the Americas
- Brugian filariasis is found in South and Southeast Asia
- Loiasis is confined to the rain forest belt of western and central Africa and equatorial Sudan

Laboratory Features

White Blood Cells

- Normal to increased
- Eosinophilia possible

Red Blood Cells

- Not remarkable

Platelets

- Not remarkable

Microfilariae in Blood May Be Seen on Stained Thick Films

- Species identification may be made by microfilaria morphology

Diagnostic Scheme

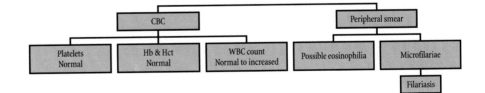

HISTOPLASMOSIS

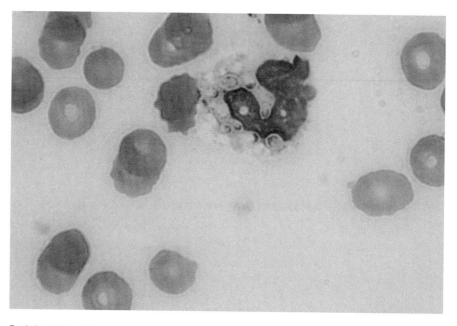

Figure II2-5   Peripheral blood smear.

Clinical Features

- Three stages
  - Acute primary
    - Asymptomatic to fever, cough, and malaise
  - Progressive disseminated
    - Hepatosplenomegaly, lymphadenopathy, or gastrointestinal ulcerations, fatigue, weakness, malaise
  - Chronic cavitary
    - Pulmonary lesions, worsening cough, dyspnea, and decreasing pulmonary function

Pathology

- Infection occurs worldwide; the endemic areas in the United States are the Ohio and Mississippi river valleys
- *Histoplasma capsulatum* is the causative agent
- Inhalation of spores in soil or dust contaminated with bird or bat droppings is the mode of exposure

Laboratory Features

White Blood Cells

■ Normal to increased

Red Blood Cells

■ Anemia in severe infections

Platelets

■ Not remarkable

Small Oval Yeast Forms May Be Seen Within Macrophages or Monocytes on Peripheral Blood, Bone Marrow, or Buffy Coat Smears

Diagnostic Scheme

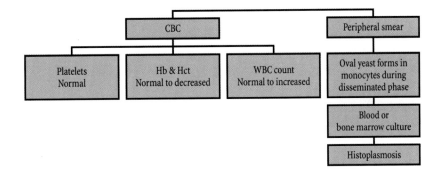

LEISHMANIASIS

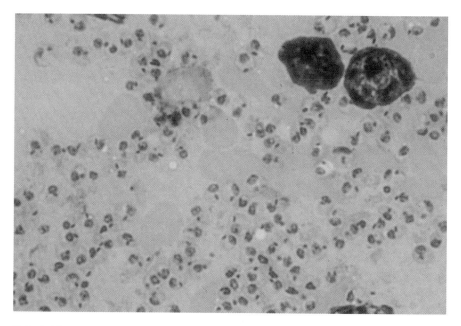

Figure II2-6   Splenic biopsy.

Clinical Features

■ Three forms exist:
  ■ Visceral leishmaniasis (kala-azar, dumdum fever)
    ■ Irregular fever, hepatosplenomegaly, and emaciation
  ■ Cutaneous leishmaniasis (oriental or tropical sore)
    ■ Sharply demarcated skin lesion at the site of infective bite
    ■ Multiple lesions are rare and take months to heal
  ■ Mucocutaneous leishmaniasis (espundia)
    ■ Primary cutaneous ulcer appears but can metastasize to nasopharyngeal
      tissue and cause gross mutilations of the nose, palate, maxillary, etc.

Pathology

- Blood and tissue flagellates that are zoonotic infections from dogs, rodents, and other reservoirs

Visceral Leishmaniasis

- Present worldwide in tropical and some temperate areas
- Caused by *Leishmania donovani* complex
- Transmitted by the bite of sandflies
- Parasites are disseminated from the skin to the lymph nodes, spleen, liver, and bone marrow
- Parasites are intracellular in macrophages
- Highly fatal without treatment

Cutaneous Leishmaniasis

- Occurs in southern Europe, Asia, Africa, the Middle East, Mexico, and Central and South America
- Causative agents are *Leishmania major, Leishmania tropica, Leishmania mexicana,* and *Leishmania braziliensis*
- Does not respond well to treatment, but once ulcers are healed, permanent immunity results

Mucocutaneous Leishmaniasis

- Caused mainly by *Leishmania viannia braziliensis*
- Parasites develop in nasopharyngeal macrophages
- Greatly feared because of gross deformities
- All forms of leishmaniasis are difficult to treat

Laboratory Features

White Blood Cells

- Leukopenia may occur in chronic forms

Red Blood Cells

- Anemia may develop in chronic forms

Platelets

- Thrombocytopenia may develop in chronic forms

The Intracellular Amastigotes May Be Seen in Stained Smears Containing Macrophages (i.e., bone marrow, splenic punctures)

- More difficult to see in cutaneous lesions

Diagnostic Scheme

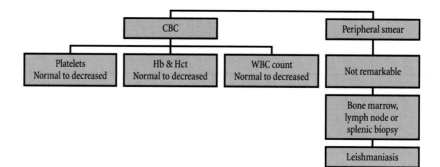

MALARIA

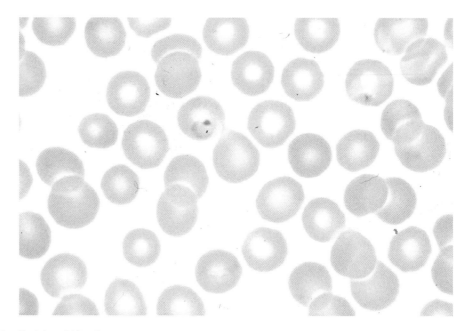

Figure II2-7   Peripheral blood smear.

Clinical Features

- Malaise, chills, and fever
- Thready pulse, headache, and nausea
- Anemia
- Jaundice
- Diarrhea
- Hepatosplenomegaly

Pathology

- Malaria is the second most important disease in the world (500 million cases per year, with 1–3 million deaths)
- Endemic in Africa, South and Southeast Asia, Central America, and northern South America
- Caused by four different species: *Plasmodium falciparum, Plasmodium vivax, Plasmodium ovale, Plasmodium malariae*
- Transmitted by the female *Anopheles* mosquitoes, which are strictly nighttime feeders

Laboratory Features

White Blood Cells

- Not remarkable

Red Blood Cells

- Hemolytic anemia

Platelets

- Not remarkable

Plasmodium *Organisms May Be Found on Thin and Thick Peripheral Blood Smears*

- Species diagnosis is made by ring-stage morphology

New Serologic Tests Are Now Becoming Available

Diagnostic Scheme

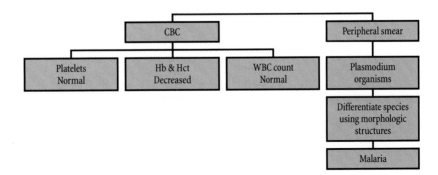

TOXOPLASMOSIS

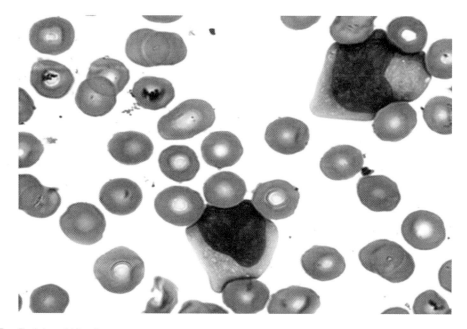

Figure II2-8   Peripheral blood smear.

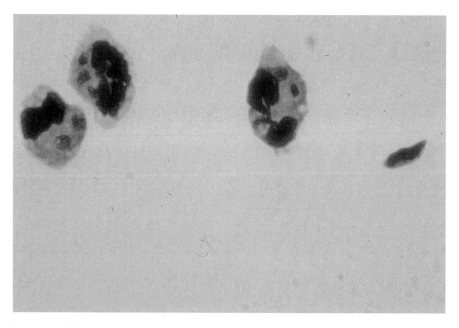

Figure II2-9   Lymph node impression.

Clinical Features

■ Usually asymptomatic
■ Principal health risk is to neonates of infected women, and it is an important cause of death in patients with AIDS
■ May cause malaise, fever, myalgia, and pharyngitis
■ Lymphadenopathy and hepatosplenomegaly
■ Severe form—pneumonitis, myocarditis, meningoencephalitis, high fever, and chills

Pathology

■ Immunocompromised patients may be at risk for a severe form of the infection
■ Caused by *Toxoplasma gondii,* which is a ubiquitous protozoan parasite of birds and mammals
■ Ingestion of oocysts from cat feces is the most common mode of oral infection
■ Undercooked meats may be infective
■ Can be transmitted transplacentally

Laboratory Features

White Blood Cells

■ Lymphocytosis
■ Atypical lymphocytes

Red Blood Cells

■ Not remarkable

Platelets

■ Not remarkable

Cluster of Tachyzoites May Be Observed in Tissue Sections or Impression Smears

■ Organisms may be seen in the white blood cells or macrophages in the bone marrow

Diagnostic Scheme

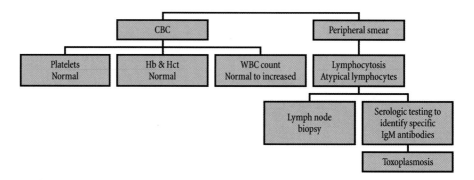

TRYPANOSOMIASIS

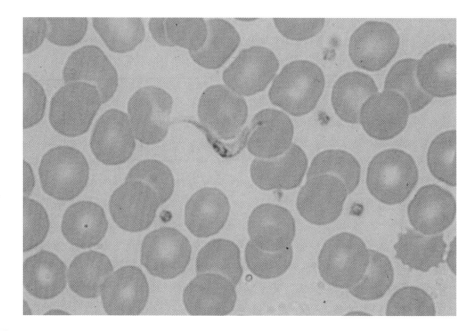

Figure II2-10

Clinical Features

African Trypanosomiasis (African Sleeping Sickness)

- Papule develops and resolves spontaneously
- Fever, headache, edematous swellings, and red rash
- Lymphadenopathy
- Central nervous system involvement—headache, personality changes, somnolence, tremor, ataxia, and coma

American Trypanosomiasis (Chagas' Disease)

- Initial infection is usually asymptomatic
- May have indurated skin lesion at the site of entry
- Fever and malaise
- Generalized lymphadenopathy and hepatosplenomegaly
- Major cause of heart disease in South America, chronic cardiomyopathy occurs in some cases

Pathology

African Trypanosomiasis

- Caused by *Trypanosoma brucei gambiense* in western and central Africa
- Caused by *Trypanosoma brucei rhodesiense* in eastern Africa
- Transmitted by tsetse flies
- May be transmitted by blood transfusion

American Trypanosomiasis

- Caused by *Trypanosoma cruzi*
- Transmitted by triatomine (reduviid) bugs
- Infected bugs deposit feces containing the organisms while feeding
- The organisms enter through the bite and invade macrophages at the site of entry
- Eventually they reach other cells of the reticuloendothelial system
- Primary damage is to neuroconductivity of the heart, esophagus, and colon
- Can be transmitted by blood transfusion

Laboratory Findings

White Blood Cells

- Not remarkable

Red Blood Cells

- Not remarkable

Platelets

- Not remarkable

Organisms May Be Observed in Thin and Thick Smears of Peripheral Blood During the Acute Phase of Infection

Diagnostic Scheme

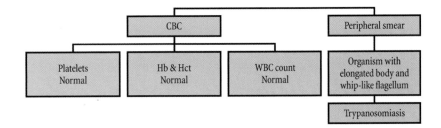

3

Reticuloendothelial System Storage Disorders

GAUCHER DISEASE

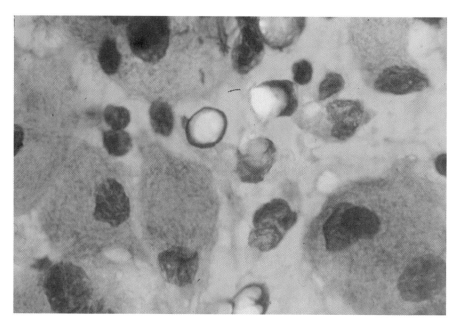

Figure II3-1   Bone marrow smear.

Clinical Features

- Splenomegaly
- Hepatomegaly
- Destruction of bone
- Pigmentation of skin in exposed areas
- Purpura and abnormal bleeding

Pathology

- Most common storage disease
- Inherited as an autosomal recessive trait
- Deficiency of beta-glucocerebrosidase
- Accumulation of glucocerebroside in macrophages of lymphoid tissue, spleen, liver, and bone marrow

Laboratory Features

White Blood Cells

■ Leukopenia ($2.0–3.0 \times 10^9$/L)
■ Relative lymphocytosis

Red Blood Cells

■ Normocytic/hypochromic anemia

Platelets

■ Moderate thrombocytopenia ($50–100 \times 10^9$/L)

Bone Marrow

■ Presence of Gaucher cells in bone marrow, spleen, and liver
  ■ Cell is large, with relatively small eccentric nucleus with coarsely clumped cytoplasm that is filled with a fibrillar pale-staining lipid

Diagnostic Scheme

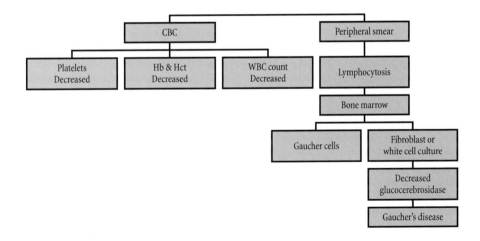

MUCOPOLYSACCHARIDOSIS

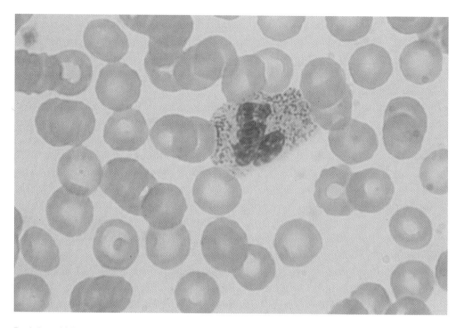

Figure II3-2   Peripheral blood smear.

Clinical Features

- Coarse facial features—flat nose and thick lips
- Skeletal abnormalities, including bone dysplasias and joint movement restriction
- Dwarfism
- Neurologic manifestations
  - Psychomotor retardation
  - Deafness
  - Ataxia
  - Mental status disturbances
- Severity varies with the type of mucopolysaccharide present
- Hepatosplenomegaly

Pathology

- A group of inherited diseases with enzyme deficiencies
- Excessive accumulation of mucopolysaccharides in body tissues
  - Arteries

- ■ Skeleton
- ■ Eyes
- ■ Joints
- ■ Skin
- ■ Liver
- ■ Bone marrow
- ■ Central nervous system
- Inherited as autosomal recessive genes with the exception of Hunter's syndrome, which is X-linked
- Depending on enzyme deficiency, different syndromes occur
  - ■ Hurler's
  - ■ Hunter's
  - ■ Sanfilippo's
  - ■ Morquio's (no Alder-Reilly inclusions seen)
  - ■ Scheie's Maroteaux-Lamy
  - ■ Sly's

Laboratory Features

White Blood Cells

- Presence of Alder-Reilly bodies in neutrophils, eosinophils, and basophils
- Inclusions may occasionally be seen in lymphocytes and monocytes

Red Blood Cells

- Not remarkable

Platelets

- Abnormally large

Diagnostic Scheme

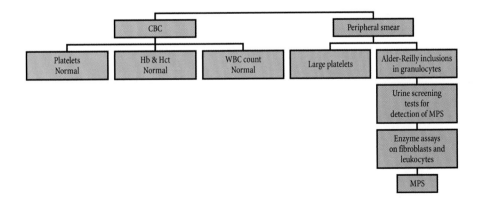

NIEMANN-PICK DISEASE

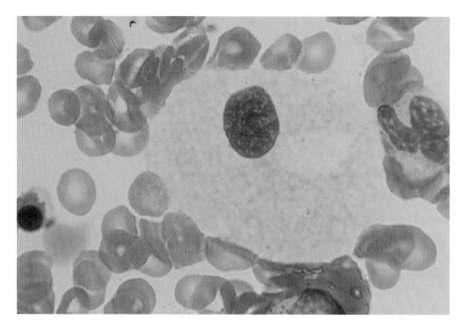

Figure II3-3   Bone marrow smear.

Clinical Features

- ■ Splenomegaly
- ■ Hepatomegaly
- ■ Severely impaired development
- ■ About one-third have a cherry-red spot on the macula of the retina
- ■ It affects girls more often than boys

Pathology

- ■ An autosomal recessive inherited disorder
- ■ Deficiency of sphingomyelinase
- ■ Accumulation of sphingomyelin in macrophages in the lymphoid system

Laboratory Features

White Blood Cells

■ Leukopenia may occur
■ Monocytes and lymphocytes may show characteristic vacuoles

Red Blood Cells

■ Mild anemia

Platelets

■ Mild thrombocytopenia

Bone Marrow

■ Finding Niemann-Pick cells in bone marrow or other tissues
  ■ These cells are filled with droplets of sphingomyelin material

Diagnostic Scheme

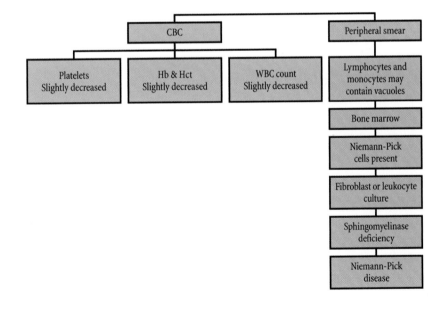

SEA-BLUE HISTIOCYTOSIS

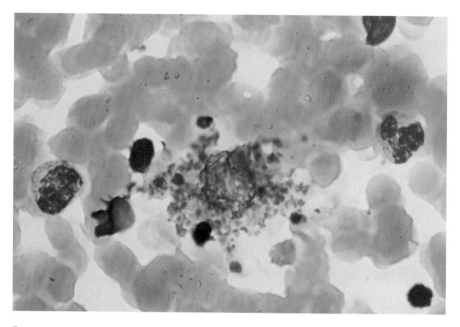

Figure II3-4   Bone marrow smear.

Clinical Features

- Splenomegaly
- Hepatomegaly
- Purpura seen in about half of the cases
- Occasional neurologic damage

Pathology

- Familial disorder in which macrophages contain blue or blue-green granules in the cytoplasm
- No specific enzyme deficiency
- Course of the disease is usually benign
- An acquired type of this disease is associated with a number of conditions

Laboratory Features

White Blood Cells

■ Not remarkable

Red Blood Cells

■ Not remarkable

Platelets

■ Normal to decreased

Bone Marrow

■ Sea-blue histiocytes are found in bone marrow and spleen
   ■ Large cells
   ■ Eccentric nucleus
   ■ Cytoplasm contains blue or blue-green granules

Diagnostic Scheme

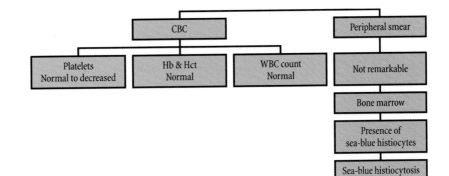

Index

Page numbers in italics followed by f denote figures; those followed by t denote tables.

A

Abnormal promyelocyte, 92, *92f*

Acanthocyte, 29, *29f*

Acanthocytosis, hereditary, 307–308, *307f, 308f*

Acid elution (Kleihauer-Betke stain), 192, *192f*

Acid phosphatase reaction
  with tartrate inhibition (TRAP), 178–179, *178f*
  without tartrate inhibition, 180, *180f*

Acquired aplastic anemia, 264–266, *264f, 266f*

Acute basophilic leukemia, 372–373, *372f, 373f*

Acute blood loss, 328–329, *328f, 329f*

Acute leukemia of ambiguous lineage (biphenotypic leukemia), 374–375, *374f, 375f*

Acute megakaryoblastic leukemia (M7), 376–378, *376f, 378f*

Acute monoblastic leukemia (M5a), 396–398, *396f, 398f*

Acute monocytic leukemia (M5b), 400–402, *400f, 402f*

Acute myelogenous leukemia with abnormal bone marrow eosinophils (M4Eo), 382–383, *382f, 383f*

Acute myelogenous leukemia with maturation (M2), 384–386, *384f, 386f*

Acute myelogenous leukemia minimally differentiated (M0), 380–381, *380f, 381f*

Acute myelogenous leukemia with multilineage dysplasia, 388–390, *388f, 390f*

Acute myelogenous leukemia without maturation (M1), 392–394, *392f, 394f*

Acute myelomonocytic leukemia (M4), 404–406, *404f, 406f*

Acute promyelocytic leukemia (M3)-hypergranular, 408–409, *408f*

Acute promyelocytic leukemia (M3)-microgranular, 410–412, *410f*

Adolescent cellularity, normal, 158, *158f*

Adult cellularity
  adult hypercellularity, 161, *161f*
  adult hypocellularity, 160, *160f*
  normal, 156, *156f*
  normal elderly cellularity, 157, *157f*

Adult T-cell lymphoma leukemia, 490–491, *490f, 491f*

Agglutination, 27, *27f*

Alder-Reilly bodies, 79, *79f*

Anemia
  acquired aplastic anemia, 264–266, *264f, 266f*
  of acute blood loss, 328–329, *328f, 329f*
  caused by myelophthisis, 262–263, *262f, 263f*
  of chronic disease, 226–227, *226f, 227f*
  chronic renal disease, 332–333, *332f, 333f*
  cold agglutinin disease, 302–303, *302f, 303f*
  congenital dyserythropoietic anemia, 268–271, *268f, 271f*
  congenital pure red blood cell aplasia, 272–273, *272f, 273f*
  Diamond-Blackfan anemia, 252–254, *252f, 254f*
  endocrine diseases, 334–335, *334f, 335f*
  erythropoietic porphyria (Gunther's Disease), 232–233, *232f, 233f*

erythropoietic protoporphyria, 234–235, *234f, 235f*

Fanconi's anemia, 274–275, *274f, 275f*

folic acid deficiency, 254–256, *254f, 256f*

glucose-6-phosphate dehydrogenase deficiency, 304–306, *304f, 306f*

hemoglobin constant spring syndrome, 236–237, *236f, 237f*

hemoglobin lepore syndrome, 238–241, *238f, 241f*

hemolytic anemias, 301–325

hereditary acanthocytosis, 307–308, *307f, 308f*

hereditary elliptocytosis, 309–311, *309f, 311f*

hereditary persistence of fetal hemoglobin, 242–244, *242f, 244f*

hereditary spherocytosis, 312–313, *312f, 313f*

hereditary stomatocytosis, 314–315, *314f, 315f*

hypochromic anemias, 219–252

hypoproliferative anemias, 261–277

immune hemolytic anemia, 316–317, *316f, 317f*

iron deficiency anemia, 245–247, *245f, 247f*

lead intoxication (plumbism), 248–249, *248f, 249f*

liver disease, 336–337, *336f, 337f*

megaloblastic anemias, 253–260

microangiopathic hemolytic anemia, 318–319, *318f, 319f*

nonimmune hemolytic anemia, 320–321, *320f, 321f*

paroxysmal nocturnal hemoglobinuria, 322–323, *322f, 323f*

Anemia (*contd.*)
    pure red cell aplasia, 276–277, *276f,*
        277f
    pyruvate kinase deficiency, 324–325,
        324f, 325f
    sideroblastic anemia, 250–252, *250f,*
        252f
    systemic disorders, anemias associated
        with, 331–339
    systemic lupus erythematosus,
        338–339, *338f, 339f*
    β thalassemia, 228–231, *228f–229f,*
        231f
    α thalassemia (3 gene deletion),
        222–223, *222f, 223f*
    α thalassemia (4 gene deletion),
        220–221, *220f, 221f*
    α thalassemia minor and silent carrier,
        224–225, *224f, 225f*
    vitamin B$_{12}$ deficiency, 258–260, *258f,*
        260f
Atypical chronic myeloid leukemia,
    478–480, *478f, 480f*
Auer rods, 80, *80f*

B

Babesiosis, 546–547, *546f, 547f*
Bands, 68–70, *68f, 69f, 70f*
    giant, 94, *94f*
Basophilia, 342–343, *342f, 343f*
Basophilic band, 70, *70f*
Basophilic megaloblast (megaloblastic
    prorubricyte), 14, *14f*
Basophilic metamyelocyte, 67, *67f*
Basophilic myelocyte, 64, *64f*
Basophilic normoblast (prorubricyte),
    6, *6f*
    and myeloblast, 144, *144f*
Basophilic stippling (punctuate
    basophilia), 47, *47f*
Basophils, 59, *59f,* 73, *73f*
Bilobed plasma cell, 124, *124f*
Biphenotypic leukemia, 374–375, *374f,*
    375f
Bite cell, 32, *32f*
Blister cell, 38, *38f*
Blood cells
    red, 3–56
    white, 57–127
Bone marrow
    cells of the reticuloendothelial system,
        167–175
    cellularity, 155–165

Borreliosis, 548–549, *548f, 549f*
Burkitt's lymphoma, 414–416, *414f, 416f,*
    522–523, *522f*
Burr cell, 34, *34f*
Butt cell, 104, *104f*

C

Cabot ring, 48, *48f*
Candidiasis, 550–551, *550f, 551f*
Cells, comparison of, 141–153
Cellularity
    adult hypercellularity, 161, *161f*
    adult hypocellularity, 160, *160f*
    erythropoiesis, 162, *162f*
    granulopoiesis, 163, *163f*
    lymphopoiesis, 164, *164f*
    megakaryopoiesis, 165, *165f*
    normal, 156–165
    normal adolescent cellularity, 158, *158f*
    normal adult cellularity, 156, *156f*
    normal elderly cellularity, 157, *157f*
    normal newborn cellularity, 159, *159f*
Chédiak-Higashi anomaly, 344–346,
    344f, 346f
Chédiak-Higashi granules, 81, *81f*
Children
    normal adolescent cellularity, 158,
        158f
    normal newborn cellularity, 159, *159f*
Chronic disease, anemia of, 226–227,
    226f, 227f
Chronic eosinophilic leukemia, 454–456,
    454f, 456f
Chronic granulomatous disease,
    348–349, *348f, 349f*
Chronic idiopathic myelofibrosis,
    458–460, *458f, 460f*
Chronic lymphocytic leukemia, 492–494,
    492f, 494f, 514–515, *514f*
Chronic lymphocytic leukemia
    lymphocyte, 109, *109f*
Chronic lymphoproliferative disorders,
    489–505
    adult T-cell lymphoma leukemia,
        490–491, *490f, 491f*
    chronic lymphocytic leukemia,
        492–494, *492f, 494f*
    hairy cell leukemia, 496–497, *496f, 497f*
    large granular lymphocytic leukemia,
        498–500, *498f, 500f*
    prolymphocytic leukemia (PLL),
        502–503, *502f, 503f*
    Sézary syndrome, 504–505, *504f, 505f*

Chronic myelogenous leukemia (CML),
    462–465, *462f, 465f*
Chronic myelomonocytic leukemia
    (CMML), 482–485, *482f, 485f*
Chronic neutrophilic leukemia, 466–467,
    466f, 467f
Chronic renal disease, 332–333, *332f, 333f*
Cleaved cell (butt cell), 104, *104f*
Codocyte (target cell), 30, *30f*
Cold agglutinin disease, 302–303, *302f,*
    303f
Comparison of cells, 141–153
Congenital dyserythropoietic anemia,
    268–271, *268f, 271f*
Congenital pure red blood cell aplasia
    (Diamond-Blackfan anemia),
    272–273, *272f, 273f*
Cytochemical stains
    acid phosphatase reaction, 178–180,
        178f, 180f
    nonspecific esterase reaction, 182–186,
        182f, 184f
    specific esterase reaction, 186–187,
        186f
    combined esterase reaction, 188–189,
        188f
    iron stain—Prussian blue reaction,
        190–191, *190f*
    acid elution (Kleihauer-Betke stain),
        192–193, *192f*
    leukocyte alkaline phosphatase stain,
        194–195, *194f*
    new methylene blue and brilliant
        cresyl blue stains, 196–197, *196f*
    periodic acid-Schiff reaction, 198–199,
        198f
    peroxidase stain, 200–201, *200f*
    sudan black B stain, 201–203, *201f*
    terminal deoxynucleotidyl transferase
        reaction, 204–205, *204f*
    toluidine blue stain, 206–207, *206f*
Cytoplasmic inclusions, 79–88

D

Dacryocyte (teardrop cell), 31, *31f*
Degmacyte (bite cell), 32, *32f*
Diamond-Blackfan anemia, 272–273,
    272f, 273f
Diffuse large B-cell lymphoma, 510–511,
    510f
Dimorphic cells, 44, *44f*
Döhle body, 82, *82f*
Drepanocyte (sickle cell), 33, *33f*

Dutcher body, 125, *125f*
Dyserythropoiesis, 56, *56f*
Dysgranulopoiesis, 93, *93f*

E
Early myelocyte, late myelocyte and, 152, *152f*
Echinocyte (burr cell), 34, *34f*
Elderly, the, normal elderly cellularity, 157, *157f*
Elliptocyte, 37, *37f*
Elliptocytosis, hereditary, 309–311, *309f*, *311f*
Endocrine diseases, 334–335, *334f*, *335f*
Eosinophilia, 350–351, *350f*, *351f*
Eosinophilic band, 69, *69f*
Eosinophilic metamyelocyte, 66, *66f*
Eosinophilic myelocyte, 63, *63f*
Eosinophils, 59, *59f*, 72, *72f*
    acute myelogenous leukemia with abnormal bone marrow eosinophils (M4Eo), 382–383, *382f*, *383f*
Erythrocytes, 4–10, *4f*
    iron-deficient, 25, *25f*
Erythrocytosis
    polycythemia vera, 210–213, *210f*, *213f*
    relative polycythemia (Gaisbock Syndrome), 214–215, *214f*, *215f*
    secondary polycythemia, 216–218, *216f*, *218f*
Erythroleukemia (M6a), 418–420, *418f*, *420f*
Erythropoiesis, 162, *162f*
Erythropoietic porphyria (Gunther's Disease), 232–233, *232f*, *233f*
Erythropoietic protoporphyria, 234–235, *234f*, *235f*
Essential thrombocythemia, 468–470, *468f*, *470f*
Esterase reaction, combined, 188, *188f*
Esterase reaction, nonspecific
    with fluoride inhibition, 182–183, *182f*
    without fluoride inhibition, 184–185, *184f*
Esterase reaction, specific, 186–187, *186f*

F
Faggot cell, 83, *83f*
Fanconi's anemia, 274–275, *274f*, *275f*
Fetal hemoglobin, hereditary persistence of, 242–244, *242f*, *244f*
Filariasis, 552–553, *552f*, *553f*
Flaming plasma cell, 126, *126f*

Fluoride inhibition
    nonspecific esterase reaction with, 182–183, *182f*
    nonspecific esterase reaction without, 184–185, *184f*
Folic acid deficiency, 254–256, *254f*, *256f*
Follicular lymphomas, 520–521, *520f*

G
Gaisbock Syndrome, 214–215, *214f*, *215f*
Gaucher cell, 170, *170f*
Gaucher disease, 570–571, *570f*, *571f*
Giant myelocytes, metamyelocytes, and bands, 94, *94f*
Giant platelet, 135, *135f*
Glucose-6-phosphate dehydrogenase deficiency, 304–306, *304f*, *306f*
Granulocytes, malignant, 89–92
Granulopoiesis, 163, *163f*
Grape cell, 127, *127f*

H
Hairy cell, 110, *110f*
Hairy cell leukemia, 496–497, *496f*, *497f*
Heinz bodies, 49, *49f*
Hematologic disease associated with microorganisms, 545–567
    babesiosis, 546–547, *546f*, *547f*
    borreliosis, 548–549, *548f*, *549f*
    candidiasis, 550–551, *550f*, *551f*
    filariasis, 552–553, *552f*, *553f*
    histoplasmosis, 554–555, *554f*, *555f*
    leishmaniasis, 556–558, *556f*, *558f*
    malaria, 560–561, *560f*, *561f*
    toxoplasmosis, 562–564, *562f*, *564f*
    trypanosomiasis, 566–567, *566f*, *567f*
Hematologic disorders
    miscellaneous disorders, 537–577
    red blood cell disorders, 209–339
    white blood cell disorders, 341–536
Hemoglobin, 280–282, *280f*, *282f*
    unstable hemoglobins, 298–300, *298f*, *300f*
Hemoglobin C crystals, 50, *50f*
Hemoglobin constant spring syndrome, 236–237, *236f*, *237f*
Hemoglobin D, 284–285, *284f*, *285f*
Hemoglobin E, 286–287, *286f*, *287f*
Hemoglobin E/β thalassemia, 288–289, *288f*, *289f*
Hemoglobin H disease, 222–223, *222f*, *223f*

Hemoglobin H inclusions, 51, *51f*
Hemoglobin lepore syndrome, 238–241, *238f*, *241f*
Hemoglobin S, 290–293, *290f*, *293f*
Hemoglobin S/β thalassemia, 294–295, *294f*
Hemoglobin S/C disease, 296–297, *296f*
Hemoglobin SC crystals, 52, *52f*
Hemoglobinopathies, qualitative, 260–278
Hemolytic anemias, 301–325
    cold agglutinin disease, 302–303, *302f*, *303f*
    glucose-6-phosphate dehydrogenase deficiency, 304–306, *304f*, *306f*
    hereditary acanthocytosis, 307–308, *307f*, *308f*
    hereditary elliptocytosis, 309–311, *309f*, *311f*
    hereditary spherocytosis, 312–313, *312f*, *313f*
    hereditary stomatocytosis, 314–315, *314f*, *315f*
    immune hemolytic anemia, 316–317, *316f*, *317f*
    microangiopathic hemolytic anemia, 318–319, *318f*, *319f*
    nonimmune hemolytic anemia, 320–321, *320f*, *321f*
    paroxysmal nocturnal hemoglobinuria, 322–323, *322f*, *323f*
    pyruvate kinase deficiency, 324–325, *324f*, *325f*
Hereditary acanthocytosis, 307–308, *307f*, *308f*
Hereditary elliptocytosis, 309–311, *309f*, *311f*
Hereditary persistence of fetal hemoglobin, 242–244, *242f*, *244f*
Hereditary spherocytosis, 312–313, *312f*, *313f*
Hereditary stomatocytosis, 314–315, *314f*, *315f*
Histiocyte, 162, *162f*
Histoplasmosis, 554–555, *554f*, *555f*
Hodgkin lymphoma, 508–509, *508f*, *509f*
Horn cell, 35, *35f*
Howell-Jolly body, 53, *53f*
Hypereosinophilic syndrome, 472–473, *472f*, *473f*
Hypersegmentation, 75, *75f*

Hypochromic anemias, 219–252
anemia of chronic disease, 226–227, *226f, 227f*
erythropoietic porphyria (Gunther's Disease), 232–233, *232f, 233f*
erythropoietic protoporphyria, 234–235, *234f, 235f*
hemoglobin constant spring syndrome, 236–237, *236f, 237f*
hemoglobin lepore syndrome, 238–241, *238f, 241f*
hereditary persistence of fetal hemoglobin, 242–244, *242f, 244f*
iron deficiency anemia, 245–247, *245f, 247f*
lead intoxication (plumbism), 248–249, *248f, 249f*
sideroblastic anemia, 250–252, *250f, 252f*
β thalassemia, 228–231, *228f–229f, 231f*
α thalassemia (3 gene deletion-hemoglobin H disease), 222–223, *222f, 223f*
α thalassemia (4 gene deletion), 220–221, *220f, 221f*
α thalassemia minor and silent carrier, 224–225, *224f, 225f*
Hypochromic cells, 45, *45f*
Hypoproliferative anemias, 261–277
acquired aplastic anemia, 264–266, *264f, 266f*
anemia caused by myelophthisis, 262–263, *262f, 263f*
congenital dyserythropoietic anemia, 268–271, *268f, 271f*
congenital pure red blood cell aplasia, 272–273, *272f, 273f*
Fanconi's anemia, 274–275, *274f, 275f*
pure red cell aplasia, 276–277, *276f, 277f*

I

Immune hemolytic anemia, 316–317, *316f, 317f*
Immunoblast, 105, *105f*
Inclusions, 47–55
abnormal plasma cells and, 124–128
cytoplasmic, 79–88
Infectious mononucleosis, 352–353, *352f, 353f*
Iron deficiency anemia, 245–247, *245f, 247f*

Iron-deficient basophilic normoblast (iron-deficient prorubricyte), 22, *22f*
Iron-deficient erythrocyte (hypochromic/microcytic), 25, *25f*
Iron-deficient orthochromic normoblast (iron-deficient metarubricyte), 24, *24f*
Iron-deficient polychromatophilic erythrocyte, 26, *26f*
Iron-deficient polychromatophilic normoblast (iron-deficient rubricyte), 23, *23f*
Iron-deficient pronormoblast (iron-deficient rubriblast), 21, *21f*
Iron-deficient series, 20–25, *20f*
Iron stain—Prussian blue reaction, 190–191, *190f*

J

Juvenile myelomonocytic leukemia, 486–488, *486f, 488f*

K

Keratocyte (horn cell), 35, *35f*
Kleihauer-Betke stain, 192, *192f*
Knizocyte (pinch cell), 36, *36f*

L

L_1 lymphoblast, 111, *111f*
L_2 lymphoblast, 112, *112f*
L_3 lymphoblast, 113, *113f*
Large granular lymphocyte, 106, *106f*
Large granular lymphocytic leukemia, 498–500, *498f, 500f*
Large lymphocyte, 107, *107f*
Large megakaryocyte, 136, *136f*
Large mononuclear megakaryocyte, 137, *137f*
Late myelocyte, and early myelocyte, 152, *152f*
Late polychromatophilic normoblast, and lymphocyte, 145, *145f*
LE cell, 88, *88f*
Lead intoxication (plumbism), 248–249, *248f, 249f*
Leishmaniasis, 556–558, *556f, 558f*
Leukemia
acute basophilic leukemia, 372–373, *372f, 373f*

acute leukemia of ambiguous lineage (biphenotypic leukemia), 374–375, *374f, 375f*
acute megakaryoblastic leukemia (M7), 376–378, *376f, 378f*
acute monoblastic leukemia (M5a), 396–398, *396f, 398f*
acute monocytic leukemia (M5b), 400–402, *400f, 402f*
acute myelogenous leukemia with abnormal bone marrow eosinophils (M4Eo), 382–383, *382f, 383f*
acute myelogenous leukemia with maturation (M2), 384–386, *384f, 386f*
acute myelogenous leukemia minimally differentiated (M0), 380–381, *380f, 381f*
acute myelogenous leukemia with multilineage dysplasia, 388–390, *388f, 390f*
acute myelogenous leukemia without maturation (M1), 392–394, *392f, 394f*
acute myelomonocytic leukemia (M4), 404–406, *404f, 406f*
acute promyelocytic leukemia (M3)-hypergranular, 408–409, *408f*
acute promyelocytic leukemia (M3)-microgranular, 410–412, *410f*
adult T-cell lymphoma leukemia, 490–491, *490f, 491f*
atypical chronic myeloid leukemia, 478–480, *478f, 480f*
Burkitt's lymphoma, 414–416, *414f, 416f*
chronic eosinophilic leukemia, 454–456, *454f, 456f*
chronic lymphocytic leukemia, 492–494, *492f, 494f, 514–515, 514f*
chronic myelogenous leukemia (CML), 462–465, *462f, 465f*
chronic myelomonocytic leukemia (CMML), 482–485, *482f, 485f*
chronic neutrophilic leukemia, 466–467, *466f, 467f*
erythroleukemia (M6a), 418–420, *418f, 420f*
hairy cell leukemia, 496–497, *496f, 497f*
juvenile myelomonocytic leukemia, 486–488, *486f, 488f*
large granular lymphocytic leukemia, 498–500, *498f, 500f*

non-Hodgkin's lymphomas of B-cell
origin-precursor B-lymphoblastic
leukemia/lymphoma, 512–513, *512f*
non-Hodgkin's lymphomas of B-cell
origin-small lymphocytic
lymphoma or chronic lymphocytic
leukemia, 514–515, *514f*
plasma cell leukemia, 526–528, *526f,
528f*
precursor lymphoblastic leukemia
(L1), 422–424, *422f*
precursor lymphoblastic leukemia
(L2), 426–428, *426f*
prolymphocytic leukemia (PLL),
502–503, *502f, 503f*
pure erythroid leukemia (M6b),
430–432, *430f, 432f*
Leukocyte alkaline phosphatase (LAP)
stain, 194–195, *194f*
Leukocyte disorders, nonmalignant,
341–369
Liver disease, 336–337, *336f, 337f*
Lymphoblast, 101, *101f*
Lymphoblastic lymphoma cell, 115,
115f
Lymphocytes, 100–102, *100f*
late polychromatophilic normoblast
and, 145, *145f*
malignant, 109–114
mature, 102, *102f*
monocytes and, 149, *149f*
monocytes and reactive, 148, *148f*
reactive, 103–108
Lymphocytosis, 354–358, *354f, 358f*
Lymphoma cells, 115–119
Lymphomas, 507–523
Hodgkin lymphoma, 508–509, *508f,
509f*
non-Hodgkin's lymphomas of B-cell
origin-Burkitt's lymphoma,
522–523, *522f*
non-Hodgkin's lymphomas of B-cell
origin-diffuse large B-cell
lymphoma, 510–511, *510f*
non-Hodgkin's lymphomas of B-cell
origin-follicular lymphomas,
520–521, *520f*
non-Hodgkin's lymphomas of B-cell
origin-mantle cell lymphoma
(intermediate lymphocytic
lymphoma), 518–519, *518f*
non-Hodgkin's lymphomas of B-cell
origin-mucosa-associated lymphoid

tissue lymphoma (MALT), 516–517,
516f
non-Hodgkin's lymphomas of B-cell
origin-precursor B-lymphoblastic
leukemia/lymphoma, 512–513, *512f*
non-Hodgkin's lymphomas of B-cell
origin-small lymphocytic
lymphoma or chronic lymphocytic
leukemia, 514–515, *514f*
Lymphopoiesis, 164, *164f*

M
Macrocyte
oral, 18, *18f*
size, 42, *42f*
Macrophage, 168, *168f*
Malaria, 54, *54f*, 560–561, *560f, 561f*
Malignant granulocytes, 89–92
Malignant lymphocytes, 109–114
Mantle cell lymphoma, 518–519,
518f
Mast cell, 74, *74f*
Mature lymphocyte, 96–97, *96f*
Mature red blood cell (mature
erythrocyte), 10, *10f*
May-Hegglin anomaly, 360–361, *360f,
361f*
May-Hegglin inclusion, 84, *84f*
Megakaryoblast, 131, *131f*
Megakaryocytes, 133, *133f*
abnormal megakaryocytic cells,
135–139
normal megakaryocytic maturation
series, 130–134, *130f*
Megakaryopoiesis, 165, *165f*
Megaloblastic anemias, 253–260
folic acid deficiency, 254–256, *254f,
256f*
vitamin B12 deficiency, 258–260, *258f,
260f*
Megaloblastic maturation series, 12–18,
12f, 512
basophilic megaloblast (megaloblastic
prorubricyte), 14, *14f*
megalocyte (oral macrocyte), 18, *18f*
orthochromic megaloblast
(megaloblastic metarubricyte),
16, *16f*
polychromatophilic megaloblast
(megaloblastic rubricyte), 15, *15f*
polychromatophilic megalocyte
(megaloblastic reticulocyte),
17, *17f*

promegaloblast (megaloblastic
rubriblast), 13, *13f*
Megalocyte (oral macrocyte), 18, *18f*
Metamyelocytes, 65–67, *65f, 66f, 67f*
giant, 94, *94f*
neutrophilic bands, and neutrophils,
153, *153f*
Metarubricyte, 8, *8f*
iron-deficient, 24, *24f*
megaloblastic, 16, *16f*
Microangiopathic hemolytic anemia,
318–319, *318f, 319f*
Microcyte, 43, *43f*
Micromegakaryocyte, 138, *138f*
Microorganisms, 85, *85f*
hematologic disease associated with,
545–567
Monoblast, 97, *97f*
and myeloblast, 147, *147f*
and promonocyte, 146, *146f*
Monocytes, 96–99, *96f, 99f*
and reactive lymphocyte, 148, *148f*
and lymphocytes, 149, *149f*
Monocytosis, 362–363, *362f, 363f*
Mononucleosis, 352–353, *352f, 353f*
Mott cell (grape cell), 127, *127f*
Mucopolysaccharidosis, 572–573, *572f,
573f*
Mucosa-associated lymphoid tissue
lymphoma (MALT), 516–517, *516f*
Myeloblast, 60, *60f*, 89–91, *89f, 90f, 91f*
and basophilic normoblast, 144, *144f*
and monoblast, 147, *147f*
and myelocytes, 142, *142f*, 143, *143f*
and promyelocytes, 143, *143f*
Myelocytes, 62–64, *62f, 63f, 64f*
early and late, 152, *152f*
giant, 94, *94f*
and myeloblasts, 142, *142f*, 143, *143f*
and promyelocytes, 143, *143f*
and pronormoblasts, 150, *150f*
Myelodysplastic syndromes, 433–452
myelodysplastic syndrome with
isolated del (5q-) chromosome
abnormality, 434–436, *434f,
436f*
refractory anemia, 438–440, *438f,
440f*
refractory anemia with excess blasts
(RAEB-1 and RAEB-2), 442–444,
442f, 444f
refractory anemia with ringed
sideroblasts, 446–448, *446f, 448f*

Myelodysplastic syndromes (*contd.*)
refractory cytopenia with multilineage
dysplasia, 450–452, *450f, 452f*
Myelophthisis, anemia caused by,
262–263, *262f, 263f*
Myeloproliferative diseases, 453–476
chronic eosinophilic leukemia,
454–456, *454f, 456f*
chronic idiopathic myelofibrosis,
458–460, *458f, 460f*
chronic myelogenous leukemia
(CML), 462–465, *462f, 465f*
chronic neutrophilic leukemia,
466–467, *466f, 467f*
essential thrombocythemia, 468–470,
468f, 470f
hypereosinophilic syndrome, 472–473,
472f, 473f
polycythemia vera, 474–476
Myeloproliferative/myelodysplastic
diseases, 477–488
atypical chronic myeloid leukemia,
478–480, *478f, 480f*
chronic myelomonocytic leukemia
(CMML), 482–485, *482f, 485f*
juvenile myelomonocytic leukemia,
486–488, *486f, 488f*

N

Neutropenia, 364–365, *364f, 365f*
Neutrophilia, 366–367, *366f, 367f*
Neutrophilic band, 68, *68f*
neutrophils, and metamyelocytes, 153,
153f
Neutrophilic metamyelocyte, 65, *65f*
Neutrophilic myelocyte, 62, *62f*
Neutrophils, 58, *58f*
neutrophilic bands, and
metamyelocytes, 153, *153f*
Niemann-Pick cell, 171, *171f*
Niemann-Pick disease, 574–575, *574f,
575f*
Non-Hodgkin's lymphomas of B-cell
origin-diffuse large B-cell
lymphoma, 510–511, *510f*
Non-Hodgkin's lymphomas of B-cell
origin-follicular lymphomas,
520–521, *520f*
Non-Hodgkin's lymphomas of B-cell
origin-mantle cell lymphoma
(intermediate lymphocytic
lymphoma), 518–519,
518f

Non-Hodgkin's lymphomas of B-cell
origin-mucosa-associated lymphoid
tissue lymphoma (MALT), 516–517,
516f
Non-Hodgkin's lymphomas of B-cell
origin-precursor B-lymphoblastic
leukemia/lymphoma, 512–513,
512f
Non-Hodgkin's lymphomas of B-cell
origin-small lymphocytic
lymphoma or chronic lymphocytic
leukemia, 514–515, *514f*
Nonhematopoietic cells, 173–175, *174f,
175f*
Nonimmune hemolytic anemia,
320–321, *320f, 321f*
Nonmalignant leukocyte disorders,
341–369
basophilia, 342–343, *342f, 343f*
Chédiak-Higashi anomaly, 344–346,
344f, 346f
chronic granulomatous disease,
348–349, *348f, 349f*
eosinophilia, 350–351, *350f, 351f*
infectious mononucleosis, 352–353,
352f, 353f
lymphocytosis, 354–358, *354f, 358f*
May-Hegglin anomaly, 360–361, *360f,
361f*
monocytosis, 362–363, *362f, 363f*
neutropenia, 364–365, *364f, 365f*
neutrophilia, 366–367, *366f, 367f*
Pelger-Huët anomaly, 368–369, *368f,
369f*
Nuclear segmentation, 75–78

O

Oral macrocyte, 18, *18f*
Orthochromic megaloblast
(megaloblastic metarubricyte),
16, *16f*
Orthochromic normoblast
(metarubricyte), 8, *8f*
Osteoblast, 174, *174f*
Osteoclast, 175, *175f*
Ovalocyte (elliptocyte), 37, *37f*

P

Pappenheimer body, 55, *55f*
Paroxysmal nocturnal hemoglobinuria,
322–323, *322f, 323f*
Pelger-Huët anomaly, 368–369, *368f,
369f*

Pelger-Huët cells, 76–77, *76f*
Pelgeroid cells, 78, *78f*
Periodic acid-Schiff (PAS) reaction,
198–199, *198f*
Peroxidase (POX) stain, 200–201, *200f*
Pinch cell, 36, *36f*
Plasma cell disorders, 525–536
plasma cell leukemia, 526–528, *526f,
528f*
plasma cell myeloma, 530–532, *530f,
532f*
Waldenström's macroglobinemia,
534–536, *534f, 536f*
Plasma cells, 120–123, *120f, 123f*
abnormal plasma cells and inclusions,
124–128
Plasmablast, 121, *121f*
Plasmacytes, 120–123
Plasmacytoid lymphocyte, 108, *108f*
Platelet disorder, quantitative, 537–544
Platelets, 134, *134f*
giant, 135, *135f*
Plumbism, 248–249, *248f, 249f*
Polychromatophilic cells, 46, *46f*
Polychromatophilic erythrocyte
(reticulocyte), 9, *9f*
Polychromatophilic megaloblast
(megaloblastic rubricyte), 15, *15f*
Polychromatophilic megalocyte
(megaloblastic reticulocyte), 17, *17f*
Polychromatophilic normoblast
(rubricyte), 7, *7f*
late polychromatophilic normoblast
and lymphocyte, 137, *137f*
Polycythemia vera, 210–213, *210f, 213f,*
474–476
Polymorphonuclear neutrophil, 71, *71f*
Precursor B-lymphoblastic leukemia/
lymphoma, 512–513, *512f*
Precursor lymphoblastic leukemia (L1),
422–424, *422f*
Precursor lymphoblastic leukemia (L2),
426–428, *426f*
Prolymphocyte, 114, *114f*
Prolymphocytic leukemia (PLL),
502–503, *502f, 503f*
Promegakaryocyte, 132, *132f*
Promegaloblast (megaloblastic
rubriblast), 13, *13f*
Promonocyte, 98, *98f*
and monoblast, 146, *146f*
Promyelocyte, 61, *61f*
abnormal, 92, *92f*

myeloblasts, and myelocytes, 143, *143f*
and pronormoblast, 151, *151f*
Pronormoblast (rubriblast), 5, *5f*
and myelocytes, 150, *150f*
and promyelocyte, 151, *151f*
Proplasmacyte, 122, *122f*
Prorubricyte, 6, *6f*
iron-deficient, 22, *22f*
megaloblastic, 14, *14f*
Prussian blue reaction—iron stain,
176–177, *176f*
Punctuate basophilia, 47, *47f*
Pure erythroid leukemia (M6b),
430–432, *430f, 432f*
Pure red cell aplasia, 276–277, *276f, 277f*
Pyknocyte (blister cell), 38, *38f*
Pyruvate kinase deficiency, 324–325,
324f, 325f

Q
Qualitative hemoglobinopathies,
279–300
hemoglobin, 280–282, *280f, 282f*
hemoglobin D, 284–285, *284f, 285f*
hemoglobin E, 286–287, *286f, 287f*
hemoglobin E/β thalassemia,
288–289, *288f, 289f*
hemoglobin S, 290–293, *290f, 293f*
hemoglobin S/β thalassemia,
294–295, *294f*
hemoglobin S/C disease, 296–297, *296f*
unstable hemoglobins, 298–300, *298f,
300f*
Quantitative platelet disorders, 537–544
thrombocytopenia, 538–540, *538f, 540f*
thrombocytosis, 542–544, *542f, 544f*

R
Reactive lymphocytes, 103–108, 148, *148f*
and monocytes, 148, *148f*
reactive (atypical) lymphocytes, 103,
103f
Red blood cell disorders
acute blood loss, 327–329
anemias associated with systemic
disorders, 331–339
erythrocytosis, 209–218
hemolytic anemias, 301–325
hypochromic anemias, 219–252
hypoproliferative anemias, 261–277
megaloblastic anemias, 253–260
qualitative hemoglobinopathies,
279–300

Red blood cells
abnormal maturation, 56
agglutination, 27, *27f*
coloring, 44–46
distribution, 27–28
erythrocyte series, 4–10, *4f*
inclusions, 47–55
iron-deficient maturation series,
20–25, *20f*
megaloblastic maturation series,
12–18, *12f*
normal maturation series, 4–10
rouleaux, 28, *28f*
shapes, 29–41
size, 42–43
Reed-Sternberg cell, 116, *116f*
Refractory anemia, 438–440, *438f,
440f*
Refractory anemia with excess blasts
(RAEB-1 and RAEB-2), 442–444,
442f, 444f
Refractory anemia with ringed
sideroblasts, 446–448, *446f, 448f*
Refractory cytopenia with multilineage
dysplasia, 450–452, *450f, 452f*
Relative polycythemia (Gaisbock
Syndrome), 214–215, *214f, 215f*
Reticulocyte, 9, *9f*
megaloblastic, 17, *17f*
Reticuloendothelial system, cells of the
abnormal cells, 170–172, *170f, 171f,
172f*
normal cells, 168–169, *168f, 169f*
Reticuloendothelial system storage
disorders, 569–577
Gaucher disease, 570–571, *570f, 571f*
mucopolysaccharidosis, 572–573, *572f,
573f*
Niemann-Pick disease, 574–575, *574f,
575f*
sea-blue histiocytosis, 576–577, *576f,
577f*
Reticulum cell, 169, *169f*
Rouleaux, 28, *28f*
Rubriblast, 5, *5f*
iron-deficient, 21, *21f*
megaloblastic, 13, *13f*
Rubricyte, 7–8, *7f*
iron-deficient, 23, *23f*
megaloblastic, 15, *15f*
polychromatophilic normoblast,
7, *7f*
Russell bodies, 128, *128f*

S
Schistocyte (schizocyte), 39, *39f*
Sea-blue histiocyte, 172, *172f*
Sea-blue histiocytosis, 576–577, *576f,
577f*
Secondary polycythemia, 216–218, *216f,
218f*
Segmented neutrophil
(polymorphonuclear neutrophil),
71, *71f*
Sézary cell, 117, *117f*
Sézary syndrome, 504–505, *504f, 505f*
Sickle cell, drepanocyte, 33, *33f*
Sideroblastic anemia, 250–252, *250f, 252f*
Small B lymphoma cell, 119, *119f*
Small cleaved lymphoma cell, 118, *118f*
Small lymphocytic lymphoma, 514–515,
514f
Spherocyte, 40, *40f*
Spherocytosis, hereditary, 312–313, *312f,
313f*
Stomatocyte, 41, *41f*
Stomatocytosis, hereditary, 314–315,
314f, 315f
Sudan black B (SBB) stain, 202–203,
202f
Systemic disorder, anemias associated
with, 331–339
chronic renal disease, 332–333, *332f*
endocrine diseases, 334–335, *334f*
liver disease, 336–337, *336f*
systemic lupus erythematosus,
338–339, *338f*
Systemic lupus erythematosus, 338–339,
338f, 339f

T
T-cells, adult T-cell lymphoma leukemia,
490–491, *490f, 491f*
Target cell, 30, *30f*
Tartrate inhibition (TRAP)
acid phosphatase reaction with,
178–179, *178f*
acid phosphatase reaction without,
180, *180f*
Teardrop cell, 31, *31f*
Terminal deoxynucleotidyl transferase
(TdT) reaction, 204–205, *204f*
β Thalassemia, 228–231, *228f–229f,
231f*
α Thalassemia (3 gene
deletion-hemoglobin H disease),
222–223, *222f, 223f*

α Thalassemia (4 gene deletion),
220–221, *220f, 221f*
α Thalassemia minor and silent carrier,
224–225, *224f, 225f*
Thrombocytopenia, 538–540, *538f,*
540f
Thrombocytosis, 542–544, *542f,*
544f
Toluidine blue stain, 206, *206f*
Toxic granulation, 86, *86f*
Toxoplasmosis, 562–564, *562f, 564f*
Trypanosomiasis, 566–567, *566f,*
567f
Type I myeloblast, 89, *89f*
Type II myeloblast, 90, *90f*
Type III myeloblast, 91, *91f*

U
Unstable hemoglobins, 298–300, *298f,*
300f

V
Vacuolated megakaryocyte, 139, *139f*
Vacuolization, 87, *87f*
Vitamin B$_{12}$ deficiency, 258–260, *258f,*
260f

W
Waldenström's macroglobinemia,
534–536, *534f, 536f*
White blood cell disorders
chronic lymphoproliferative disorders,
489–505
leukemias, 371–432
lymphomas, 507–523
myelodysplastic syndromes, 433–452
myeloproliferative diseases, 453–476
myeloproliferative/myelodysplastic
diseases, 477–488
nonmalignant leukocyte disorders,
341–369
plasma cell disorders, 525–536
White blood cells
abnormal maturation, 93–94
abnormal plasma cells and inclusions,
124–128
basophilic series, 59, *59f*
cytoplasmic inclusions, 79–88
eosinophilic series, 59, *59f*
lymphocyte maturation series,
100–102, *100f*
lymphoma cells, 115–119
malignant granulocytes, 89–92
malignant lymphocytes, 109–114
monocyte maturation series, 96–99,
96f
neutrophilic series, 58, *58f*
normal granulocytic maturation
series, 58–74
nuclear segmentation, 75–78
plasma cell series, 120–123,
120f
reactive lymphocytes, 103–108